D1707232

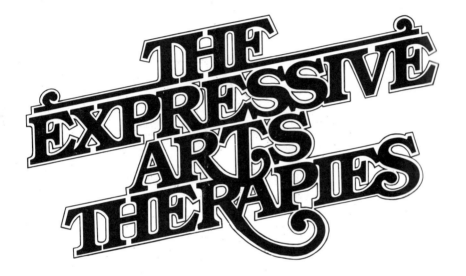

THE EXPRESSIVE ARTS THERAPIES

Elaine & Bernard Feder

A SPECTRUM BOOK

PRENTICE-HALL, INC., Englewood Cliffs, New Jersey 07632

Library of Congress Cataloging in Publication Data

Feder, Elaine.
    The expressive arts therapies.

    (A Spectrum Book)
    Includes bibliographical references and index.
    1. Art therapy. 2. Music therapy. 3. Dance
therapy. I. Feder, Bernard, joint author. II. Title.
RC489.A7F43   616.89'165   80-23887
ISBN 0-13-298059-2
ISBN 0-13-298042-8 (pbk.)

Interior design and production by
Nancy Earle
THE BOOK DEPARTMENT, INC.
52 Roland Street
Charlestown, Massachusetts 02129

Editorial/production supervision by Louise M. Marcewicz
Manufacturing buyer: Barbara A. Frick
Cover design by Graphikann

Printed in the United States of America

Prentice-Hall International, Inc., London
Prentice-Hall of Australia Pty. Limited, Sydney
Prentice-Hall of Canada, Ltd., Toronto
Prentice-Hall of India Private Limited, New Delhi
Prentice-Hall of Japan, Inc., Tokyo
Prentice-Hall of Southeast Asia Pte. Ltd., Singapore
Whitehall Books Limited, Wellington, New Zealand

Contents

Preface

In this book, we have attempted to pull together the various theories underlying the arts therapies and to see how these theories are applied in practice. This we have done in a number of ways: by asking therapists what they do, by listening to therapists talk to each other at conventions, and by reading their self-conscious statements and writings. We have examined their research studies, and we have considered their criticisms of each other, as well as their own considerable self-criticisms. But we have also tried to come as close as seemed feasible to watching what arts therapists actually do. While we would have liked to travel around the country watching therapists at work and recording what we saw and heard, we did this in a relatively small number of cases: most therapy is a private affair, and the presence of an observer in itself changes and distorts the relationships.

So we went back to asking therapists. But our focus in this connection was on the practice — the *what* — of the arts therapies. We asked therapists to talk about cases, and we searched the literature to find the cases that therapists thought were worth discussing. Of these, we have selected some to present in vignette form. We must caution, however, against the tendency to interpret these anecdotal situations as models of treatment methods, or as approaches to be emulated. Nor are they thumbnail case histories designed to provide evidence of the relative effectiveness of various types of treatment. Anecdotal data of this nature, especially in isolated and specific situations, are rarely considered compelling evidence to support outcome claims. The case histories and descriptions of sessions are attempts to flesh out the abstract discussion of theory by providing snapshots of therapists at work. They provide views of the ways some therapists work and of the things some therapists do in applying theoretical principles. Moreover, no single case shows more than an individual therapist's approach to a specific problem at a specific time. While a single case history or session may provide some clues about a therapist's philosophy, it cannot capture or encapsulate that philosophy.

We owe a debt of gratitude to those therapists who agreed to share with us — and with you — glimpses of their work, often at considerable expense of time and effort. More than one therapist remarked on the pain and difficulty of writing about therapy, in contrast with doing it. And to our contributors we owe an apology. The giant Procrustes of Greek mythology used his iron bedstead as the measure of all travelers who fell into his hands; those who were too short were stretched to size, and those who were too tall had their limbs chopped off. To many of our contributors, our editing of their cases to vignette length might well have appeared Procrustean.

We were impressed with the openness with which most of those we approached for contributions or for comments were willing to discuss their philosophies, their methodologies, and their experiences. The case contributors to whom we make particular and grateful acknowledgment are Myra Levick, A.T.R., Dianne Dulicai, D.T.R., and Cynthia Briggs, R.M.T., all of Hahneman Medical College in Philadelphia; Helen Landgarten, A.T.R., and Dr. Beth Kalish, D.T.R., both of Loyola Marymount University in Los Angeles; Sister Mariam Pfeifer, R.M.T., I.H.M., of St. Joseph's Children's and Maternity Hospital, Scranton, Pennsylvania; Arlynne Stark, D.T.R., of Goucher College, Towson,

Maryland; Liljan Espenak, D.T.R., of the New York Medical College and the Alfred Adler Mental Health Clinic, New York City; Berti Klein of Academia Nacional de la Danza, Cuernavaca, Mexico and Dr. Hella Moller, a child psychologist in private practice in Sarasota, Florida.

Our debt extends to many others. The ideas in this book grew out of interactions with arts therapists, psychiatrists, psychotherapists, research psychologists, scholars in a variety of disciplines, and practicing and performing artists, all of whom provided insights into the structure of the arts, or of the therapies, and the ways in which the underlying theories converge. Talking to us about their own music, for example, pianist Leonid Hambro, flutist Samuel Baron, and violinist Joseph Silverstein dealt repeatedly with some of the principles that underlie music therapy. While we are obligated to all of those who shared with us their time, their knowledge, and the fruits of their experience, space limitations do not permit us to name them all. In particular, however, we must offer special thanks to Irmgard Bartenieff, Dr. Judith S. Kestenberg, Dr. Paul C. Trieloff, and to new college faculty members: Dr. Marion Hoppin, Dr. Ronald Riddle, and especially to Gail Mead, who provided vital encouragement and active support in the critical early stages of the work.

I

From Time
Immemorial

The use of the expressive arts in therapy can be traced in time to the dim beginnings of human artistic expression; it can be tracked across the continents and found in virtually every human culture. The evidence is available in artifacts and pictograms, in analogous customs and ways of primitive peoples today, and in scattered historical records.

BEFORE THE DAWN OF HISTORY

During the late stages of the Old Stone Age, we encounter the earliest works of art known to us. The evidence suggests strongly that to primitive peoples the visual arts were functional rather than aesthetic. They were used purposefully — in magical incantation, in invocation of the spirits, in exorcism. That so many of the early

1

works of art were hidden in the bowels of the earth, deep in underground caves, suggests that they served purposes other than mere decoration. Our knowledge of the psychology of humans, coupled with our increasing body of data about primitive peoples, suggests that among other highly practical functions—such as providing places for evil spirits to rest, ensuring success in the hunt, "creating" animals when game was scarce, and invoking rain or fertility—art was used to treat physical and mental disorders. This inference is supported by the nature of primitive art. Says Sigfried Giedion, "Primitive art, in contrast to our own directly inherited tradition in art, is never naturalistic. There is no naturalistic art in prehistory."[1]

We have no direct knowledge about whether Paleolithic humans danced, but we do know that Neolithic people did, because we have evidence from cave paintings and artifacts that date back to this period. While we do know that dance existed, however, we do not know what it looked like in terms of its quality as dance, as movement rather than position. But rhythmic movement, perhaps accompanied by sound and using the body itself as an instrument, was surely one of the earliest forms of self-expression, in which humans related their own beings to the constantly changing world in which they lived, a world filled with the rhythm of movement, of the days, and of the seasons.

Again, using as a base our knowledge derived from anthropology, we can infer that, just as early art was probably not focused on decoration, early dance was more than mere self-enjoyment. Among primitive peoples today, dance is religious, self-expressive, and communicative. Dance historian Walter Sorell writes that to primitive people, dance is never superficial or without purpose: "It is not done because it 'is the thing to do,' but because it 'is' the thing."[2] The primitive !Kung tribesmen of the Kalahari Desert today include everyone in the healing dance, according to psychologist-anthropologist Richard Katz, "for in healing, the !Kung make no distinction among their physical, emotional and spiritual needs."[3] The healing energy comes from the gods, and the dances and songs heat up the energy to facilitate the healing process.

In the area of music, as with dance, we have no direct evidence, but it is reasonable to infer that it, too, was used for incantation, magic, prayer, and therapy. Our evidence is limited to analogy and artifacts that point to the existence of instruments for making music; of the music itself, there is no record. We have pictures of a soundbox of a harp from Ur that has been dated at about 2600 BC,[4] but the sound of the music must remain forever lost from the time before AD 1000. Only at that late date were notation systems devised to reconstruct the sound of musical compositions.[5]

Inferences about the use of music as therapy during prehistoric times are strengthened by the knowledge that it is used today for that purpose by primitive peoples. In some parts of Africa, the medicine man still uses a magic drum and an *Ouombi* harp to play over the stomach of a patient, and in the Indian tribes of Ontario, magicians and shamans are also music teachers.[6] In *Our Musical Heritage*, Curt Sachs points out that in every part of the world, music (and musical instruments) served magical rather than aesthetic purposes:

> The instruments . . . are meaningful, not attractive or beautiful. Their significant sounds, as soft or strong or muffled or shrill; their outer shapes, as round or pointed; their colors, as lifeless white or bloody red; their very motion, as striking, stamping, scraping, or rubbing — they all entangle the early instruments in an intricate maze of pre-musical, magical connotations, far from aesthetic pleasure. Both as objects and as sound-emitters, the instruments stand for the mystic realms of the sun and the moon, for the all-creative male and female principles, for fertility, rain, and wind; and they act as the strongest charms at man's disposal when he performs the vital rites of magic to protect his health and existence.[7]

A good deal is known about the use of music, dance, and art among the Indians of North America, from which we may reasonably infer the widespread use of such therapies among other preliterate peoples. The Navajo, for example, in their well-known "curing" sings, use combinations of song, dance, and sandpainting, in which specific patterns are used for specific illnesses.[8] John Collier, former commissioner of Indian affairs, writes that "a Navajo sing is communal healing, and the sick patient throws the healing back to all who are assisting him, in a profound process of therapeutic suggestion and self-suggestion which reaches to the obscure, central deeps of the body and the soul."[9] Central elements of the singing cure are ceremonial dances and the dry paintings, or sandpaintings, which are almost exclusively symbolic and bring to mind Jung's archetypal images.

EGYPTIANS, GREEKS, AND HEBREWS

From the earliest records available to us, we know that the historic ancients used the arts — particularly music — in the treatment of physical and mental problems. The ancient Egyptian priest-physicians referred to music as "the physic of the soul" and recorded their chant-therapies on the famous medical *papyri.*[10] The Bible takes note of the therapeutic value of music: "And whenever the evil spirit . . . came upon Saul, David would take the lyre and play with his hand and Saul would be relieved and feel restored and the evil spirit would depart from him."[11]

The Greeks, who early understood the relationship between mind and body and soul, saw clearly the link between music and medicine. Apollo was simultaneously the god of music and the physician of the gods, commonly called Alexikakos, the averter of ills. Apollo's son Aesculapius became the god of medicine. His other son, Orpheus, first among mortal musicians, was credited with mysteries and cures; his playing could soothe savage beasts. The touching legend of Orpheus testifies to the power of music, even over the underworld. The temples of Aesculapius were healing shrines as well as temples of worship, and in attendance were hymn specialists, called *aretalogists*, as well as priests.[12] Aesculapius himself prescribed music for the emotionally disturbed.[13]

The Greeks, however, made use of music as therapy in the rational as well as the mystic domain. Plato considered music a "medicine of the soul." In keeping with the Greek search for order in all things, it was natural that music should be viewed as an ordering, as well as an aesthetic, discipline; in fact, it was commonly associated with mathematics. When the soul had lost its harmony, Plato said, melody and rhythm assist in restoring it to order and concord.[14] Aristotle, that careful observer of human nature, identified as a benefit of music the function of "emotional catharsis." He asserted that persons who suffer from uncontrollable emotions, "after listening to melodies which raise the soul to ecstasy, relapse to their normal conditions as if they had experienced a medical or purgative treatment."[15]

The Greek belief in music as a rational ordering system was widespread, at least among the educated. Even Democritus, who first suggested that all matter is composed of atoms (and who is generally considered a staunch materialist), assumed the existence of some kind of soul to vitalize the material body and believed in the regulation of the body through rhythmic principles.[16] Engaging in extensive music therapy, Pythagoras, the mathematician–physician, used dance and music with mental patients. He introduced a theory of psychobiosis, in which music (which he called "musical medicine") played a central role in promoting order, proportion, and measure. Indeed, according to Bruno Meinecke, Pythagoras deserves to be known as "The Father of Psychotherapeutics."[17]

It might be noted that the Greek use of music in therapy seems to have focused on listening to music, rather than making it. Although Aristotle advocated the use of musical rattles as an outlet for the pent-up energies of otherwise destructive children,[18] the major historical references seem to be on the calming effects of listening to music. Music historian Henry Sigerist writes: "When a disorder had developed, the Greek physician tried to restore the lost balance physically with medicine, mentally with music."[19]

Medical practitioners among the Greeks were apparently as cautious about the overuse of popular therapeutic practices as are many physicians today. Caelius Aurelianus condemned the indiscriminate use of music after observing that "in the treatment of madness, certain physicians employ exciting music without any discretion which may provoke good effects when applied the right way, but on the other hand may cause much harm in a number of cases."[20]

For the Greeks, dance was apparently a preventive more than it was a cure of illness or disorder; it was seen as a means of achieving health in every part of the individual.[21] To the Greeks, who saw order in all the universe, the term *disorder*, whether applied to the physical or the mental, was probably meant much more literally than it is today. The Greek approach to preventive medicine could be conceptualized as the interrelationship of mind, body, and soul in balanced harmony.

This Greek ideal of balance is one we still admire — at least in principle. The great national games at Olympia, Delphi, Corinth, and Nemea, and the myriad local festivals, all included, in addition to the usual athletic contests, competitions in drama, music, and poetry. The great gymnasium at Pergamum contained not only tracks, fields, and baths, but a small theater for practicing oratory and studios for painting and sculpture.[22]

Even during the Golden Age of Greece, however, the strains of increasing competition and the pressures to win were creating cracks that were to result eventually in a split between body and mind. The games were invented by aristocrats who cultivated knowledge, art, and prowess for honorific or sacred purposes rather than for practical or productive ones. The bribery, cheating, and professionalism that were coming to mark the competitions were merely manifestations of the growing materialism that the intellectuals deplored. Xenaphon, who attacked the coarse, brute strength of body, was repelled even by the earthiness of Zeus, who could not live down his lusty youth; he chose to recast the king of the gods as incorporeal.[23] Plato rejected the crass materialism of the Milesian philosophers and distinguished between the realm of the physical and the mundane and that of the pure and the abstract, which he much preferred.

THE BODY-MIND SCHISM
OF THE MIDDLE AGES

By the Middle Ages, Plato's distinction had been raised to the order of dogma by generations of Christian theologians, who reviled and chastised the human body. Thomas Aquinas argued that man had the mind of an angel imprisoned in the body of an animal; to Thomas à Kempis, the body was a "dung heap"; and St. Francis called it "poor brother donkey."

The arts occupied an ambiguous position. On the one hand, music and the visual arts were pressed into the service of God. The Abbot Suger, for example, arguing that we could come to understand absolute beauty — God — only through the effects of beautiful objects on our senses, turned the royal Abbey of St. Denis into a virtual jewel box.[24] On the other hand, profane music — and certainly dance — was seen as an instrument of Satan; throughout Europe, we find legends, such as those of the Pied Piper and the red shoes, that testify to the power for evil that music and dance contained. Dance historian Walter Sorell sees the Church's opposition to dancing as an application of St. Paul's contempt for the body and its functions.[25] Even with regard to the lowly body, however, an ambivalence is evident; for example, the kings of France and England had been granted the divine power to cure certain diseases by "the laying on of hands."[26]

Perhaps the most dramatic evidence of this ambivalence is the Church's grudging acceptance of dance in legitimizing what it could not prevent. In doing so, the Church unwittingly aided in the development of Italy's best-known folk dance, the *tarantella*. A disease that had been prevalent in Italy, *tarantism*, had always been attributed to the sting of the tarantula. The illness, which persists to this day, normally occurs in the summer at harvest time. It is characterized by alternating seizures of uncontrollable physical frenzy and complete inertia, withdrawal, or prostration. The only cure was catharsis, which could be obtained by dance, music, and the use of symbolic colors. According to some authorities, such convulsive dances were actually nervous disorders, essentially neuroses, that were known throughout Europe under a variety of names:

St. Vitus' Dance, the Dancing Mania, the Dance of St. Joan, St. John's Dance, Tanzplage, Orchestromania, and the Lascivious Dance.[27] Sorell speculates that Hans Christian Anderson's story of the red shoes may be based on a variant form of the same phenomenon. Sigerist believes that the dancing mania in southern Italy was a persistence of ancient rites; he writes that the Church

> could not assimilate the orgiastic rites of the cult of Dionysos (which the people of Apulia had practiced for many centuries) but had to fight them. And yet these very rites that appealed to the most elementary instincts were the most deeply rooted. They persisted, and we can well imagine that the people gathered secretly to perform the old dances and all that went with them. In doing so they sinned, until one day . . . the meaning of the dance had changed. The old rites appeared as symptoms of a disease. The music, the dance, all that wild orgiastic behavior were legitimized. . . . The people who indulged in these exercises were no longer sinners but the poor victims of the tarantula.[28]

Whether neurosis, mass hysteria, or affliction attributable to an ancient and persistent rite, tarantism called for a treatment that was basically dance therapy: dancing to the music that came to be known as the tarantella.[29] In most of southern Italy, the tarantella has come to be a folk dance in a variety of forms, but some observers have found, in isolated parts of the region, tarantella rites that obviously follow the ancient pattern. Ernesto de Martino, describing such rites, calls the musicians "music therapists in the full sense of the words." They know the illness and its symptoms; they know the music from which the appropriate tunes are to be chosen. They must find the music that is acceptable to the spider that has taken possession of the patient, and they must organize their playing according to the four stages of the disease: sting, possession by the spider and identification with the movements appropriate to that spider, return of identity to the patient, and, finally, the fight against the spider.[30]

The musicians must explore the various kinds of music to reveal the particular kind of spider that has taken possession. The dancing tarantula needs stimulation by rapid music, the effect of which is stimulated by green ribbons and accoutrements. The violent, aggressive tarantula responds to rousing rhythms and to the color red. The sleeping spider evokes inertia, while the sad and melancholic spider, spurred by brown, needs dismal, sad music to dance.[31]

In retrospect, it is not easy to ascertain the degree to which the dancing mania throughout Europe parallels modern forms of mental disorder. Some of the victims of modern tarantism have been diagnosed as schizophrenic or manic.[32] It is hard to believe, however, that all of the victims of the dancing illnesses were psychotic. What is more likely is that the dancing craze itself was a reflection of the time. Charles W. Hughes reports that the victims of the dance mania suffered from melancholia and depression.[33] When we consider that during the period, the Black Death was sweeping Europe and that the population of Europe as a whole is estimated to have declined from about sixty to about thirty-five million, the terror, the depression, and the feeling of utter helplessness that pervaded Europe may well have resulted in mass neurosis on a truly grand scale.

THE RENAISSANCE OF THE ARTS IN THERAPY

Throughout the Middle Ages, the practice of medicine in Europe consisted largely of prayer, incantation, exorcism, bleeding, and crude surgery. In the Islamic world, on the other hand, scholars had rediscovered the works of the ancient Greek philosophers and mathematicians. In medicine, the Arabic and Jewish physicians, like the Greeks, saw the body and the soul as intertwined. Both were subject to the laws of nature that frequently were described in mathematical and musical terms. Like the Greeks, the scholars of the Islamic world, seeking order and regularity, looked for the connections that held the universal system together. The rotation of the heavenly bodies, variations in mood, and changes in pulse rate, for example, were manifestations of the same order and were related to each other.

Integral to this universal order was musical regularity. The universe itself moved in terms of seven whole notes, which were approximated by the tones of the musical scale. Music, therefore, represented order and played an important part in medicine. In Cairo, to which the earliest known hospitals in the Western tradition can be traced, music was played continually in the wards; human voices and stringed instruments were chosen in proper proportion to the universal order.[34]

It was not until well after the Crusades that the Europeans rediscovered the ancients — a rediscovery that came largely through the work of Moslem and Jewish scholars. Not only did the Western world retrieve the works of the ancient Greek thinkers through Islam, but Europeans adopted the interpretations given this material by the Arabs. In the fourteenth century, the only explanation of Aristotle's work permitted at the University of Paris was that of Averroës, a scholar of twelfth-century Spain.[35]

The European Renaissance of the fourteenth and fifteenth centuries was marked by a widespread revival of interest, first in classical literature, then in the artistic and medical ideas of the ancients. The legacy from the past was hailed and adopted, often uncritically, and often colored by Islamic interpretation. The medical encyclopedia compiled in the eleventh century by the Moslem, Avicenna, was a standard reference work in Europe until the middle of the seventeenth century.

Nevertheless, the time was one of social grace and creative energy; learned and inquiring individuals pursued their investigations into numerous fields, eschewing a narrow specialization. Because so many physicians of the day were music lovers and music players, it was natural that the Greek beliefs about the relationships between music and health should hold special interest for them. In particular, the theory of Empedocles, a physician and philosopher of the fifth century BC, underlays a good deal of Renaissance medical thought. Empedocles had suggested that the universe is made up of four elements: earth, air, fire, and water. These four elements had their counterparts in the four humors of Hippocrates — the fluids entering into the constitution of the body: blood, phlegm, yellow bile and black bile. It was only a matter of time before these humors were correlated with personality types: sanguine, phlegmatic, choleric, and melancholic. It is fascinating that during the Renaissance, the four cosmic elements were assigned their musical counterparts as well: bass, tenor, alto, and soprano. Physicians of the time conjectured widely on the relationships between the humors and music.[36]

The Renaissance awe of classical civilization was the impetus for a renewed interest in the arts therapies, especially in the medical use of music. Virtually every physician of the period was familiar with the classical sources, particularly Pythagoras. Unfortunately, as has been mentioned, the physicians of the time tended to accept the Greek authorities uncritically, and their expectations colored their observations. We read about music that chases pestilence, banishes madness, eradicates drunkenness, and cures a multitude of ills. The great surgeon Ambroise Paré writes of the cure of spider bites and the relief of sciatica and gout, saying that "music gives ease to pain." One of the chapters of Paré's major medical work — a chapter in which he discusses the effects of music listening — is entitled, "Of Certain Wonderful and Extravagant Ways of Curing Diseases."[37]

Like the Greeks, the physicians of the Renaissance appreciated the effects of music on an individual's state of mind and its value in preventive medicine. In the *Fasciculo di Medicina* of 1493, readers are warned to guard against anger, sorrow, fear, worry, and cogitation. (Given the prevalence of the epidemic plagues of the fourteenth and fifteenth centuries, it is easy to understand the assumption that too much thinking could be bad for your health.) Instead, readers are urged to make merry and enjoy themselves "with music, reading of stories, and the like."[38] And in his advice against plague, Tommaso del Garbo discusses the importance of a happy state of mind, a condition to which listening to music is an important contributor.[39]

The major value of music in medicine lay in its use as a cathartic and in its calming influence, especially in the treatment of mental disorders. In his extraordinary book, *The Anatomy of Melancholy*, physician Robert Burton wrote that "besides that excellent power [music] hath to expel many other diseases, it is a sovereign remedy against Despair and Melancholy, and will drive away the Devil himself."[40]

With the Scientific Revolution following hard on the heels of the Renaissance, a more orderly approach emerged to the investigation of the arts in medicine. As during the Renaissance, the emphasis was on music; during the eighteenth century, an increasing number of physicians noted and investigated the purely physiological effects of music, particularly the relationships between bodily and musical rhythms, and between pulse and musical beat. They observed the effects of music on breathing, blood pressure, and digestion, as well as on mood.[41] The old claims of miracle cures and the argument that music is a general panacea were subjected to critical appraisal. For example, Luigi Desbout, surgeon of the Royal Regiment of Tuscany, after describing a cure of hysteria with music, remained cautious about generalizing; he urged a serious study of the relation of music to disease and suggested the reasoned use of music in the treatment of hysterical, convulsive, and hypochondriac diseases.[42]

The state of thinking about the arts in therapy during the eighteenth century is illustrated by the work of Louis Roger, a physician of Montpellier, France. In his work, one of the better books of the period, Roger rejected much of the work on music and medicine that had been done in the past, on the ground that little of it was based on observation or experiment. His own treatise, based on case histories that had been carefully observed and recorded, resulted in a psychology of musical enjoyment. The elements of his theory, however, were not very different from those of the Greeks. Like the Greeks, he saw music as a natural ordering device that appealed to the mind's craving for structure — a theory that presages much of Gestalt psychological theory. In terms of its effects on the body itself, Roger sought a mechanical relationship. He saw the body's nervous system, on which music acted through sympathetic vibrations, as made up largely of fluids and gases. Listening to pleasant music, Roger asserted, was salutary, because the music would stimulate the vibration of the nerves and help them to throw off the thickened and foreign humors that had attached themselves to the nerves.[43]

By the end of the eighteenth century, the work on the arts in therapy consisted largely of a rather impressive collection of carefully noted observations — largely on the effects of music on the body — and a host of bizarre conclusions drawn from these observations.

THE VICTORIAN DEBASEMENT
OF THE BODY

The eighteenth century had been known to the intellectuals of the time as the *Age of Enlightenment*. To the degree that a frank and unabashed recognition of the human body and its functions are concerned, it was indeed an age of enlightenment. In contrast, the English and American Victorians of the next century subjected the body to a debasement that may be unparalleled in history. Not only was the body itself denied and banished from speech and sight, but words and objects that even suggested the body were transformed. Captain Frederick Marryat, an English novelist, remarked on a piano he saw in a young ladies' seminary in New York State with its legs covered by frilly, little pantaloons. In Cincinnati, Hiram Powers, possibly the best-known American sculptor of the time, was forced to dress his nude statue, *The Greek Slave*, in a calico blouse and flannel drawers. When Powers exhibited his *Chanting Cherubs* in Boston, the cherubs were required to wear pants.[44]

Not only the body, but even feelings that emanated from the body were resolutely suppressed. Sylvester Graham, a lay preacher who is best known today for the fact that he invented the graham cracker, delivered and printed a remarkable series of lectures. "When we are *conscious* that we have a stomach or a liver from any *feeling* in these organs," Graham asserted, "we may be certain that something is wrong." The sex act, to Graham, was a trauma that could be justified only by overwhelming need. The consequence of too much sex (more than once a month) included a long list of diseases, from impaired vision to loss of memory.[45]

In all fairness, it should be pointed out that this debasement of the body was a vulgar or popular phenomenon. Victorian intellectuals, including Thomas Carlyle, Charles Kingsley, John Stuart Mill, and John Ruskin, to name a few, held a remarkably modern view of the interdependence of body and mind. In fact, to such Victorian thinkers, rest cures, "taking the waters," and mountain climbing were more than merely therapeutic methods for maintaining or restoring physical health; they involved a complex relationship between humans and the universe they inhabited. And these thinkers, profoundly influenced by the rapidly developing sciences of physiology and physiological psychology, tended to view body-mind in holistic terms. In fact, Carlyle and his disciple Kingsley saw the body as the temple of the spirit.[46]

Such views, however, were hardly representative of the popular thinking of the time, especially among the middle classes, who regarded references to the body, in a peculiar perversion of the term, as "vulgar." That the mind-body dichotomy has not yet disappeared is documented by the fact that the *Encyclopedia of Philosophy* still has no reference under "body." One cross-reference appears under "body-mind problem" on page 328 of the 1967 edition and refers the reader to an article in which the order is corrected to "mind-body problem."

THE REEMERGENCE OF THE ARTS IN THERAPY

The rediscovery of the body and the reemergence of the arts in the treatment of disorders can be attributed in large part to the development of modern psychotherapy. This rediscovery of the body can easily be overstated; as we shall see in the next chapter, the bulk of psychotherapy is still verbal and still rests on the implicit assumption that the psyche resides in the head and must be approached in the language of the head — words. The old distinctions between psyche and soma still prevail, for the most part, and the old hierarchies still rule. The relationship between mind and body is acknowledged in modern medicine, but is almost always expressed as psychosomatic, rather than somatopsychic.

Nevertheless, the recognition of the relationship itself made it almost inevitable that the modern psychotherapies would acknowledge the role of the nonverbal in the therapeutic process. However, the dominant psychotherapeutic theories have shaped the direction in which modern arts therapies have developed. What has emerged as the expressive therapies represents a cross-fertilization of theory and practice from both the artistic fields themselves and from the essentially verbal psychotherapies. In the next chapter, we shall examine the basic groups of psychotherapies and explore some of the implications for the arts therapies.

REFERENCE NOTES

1. S. Giedion, *The Eternal Present: The Beginning of Art* (New York: Pantheon Books, 1962), p. 18.
2. Walter Sorell, *The Dance Through the Ages* (New York: Grosset and Dunlap, 1967), p. 10.
3. Richard Katz, "The Painful Ecstasy of Healing," *Psychology Today* 10, no. 7 (December, 1976):81.
4. H. W. Janson and Joseph Kerman, *A History of Art and Music* (Englewood Cliffs, N.J.: Prentice-Hall, and New York: Harry N. Abrams, n.d.), p. 15.
5. Ibid., p. ix.
6. Juliette Alvin, *Music Therapy* (New York: Basic Books, 1975).
7. Curt Sachs, *Our Musical Heritage*, 2nd ed. (Englewood Cliffs, N.J.: Prentice-Hall, 1955), p. 3.
8. Peter Farb, *Man's Rise to Civilization as Shown by the Indians of North America from Primeval Times to the Coming of the Industrial State* (New York: E. P. Dutton, 1968), p. 238; Ira Moskowitz and John Collier, *American Indian Ceremonial Dances* (New York: Crown Publishers, Inc., Bounty Books, 1972), p. 57.
9. Moskowitz and Collier, *American Indian Ceremonial Dances*, p. 40.
10. Felix Marti-Ibañez, "Psychic Muse: Music, the Dance, and Medicine," *MD* 20, no. 10 (October, 1976):13.
11. 1 Sam. 16:23
12. Alvin, *Music Therapy*, p. 30.
13. S. Clark, *Psychiatry Today* (Baltimore: Penguin Books, 1971).
14. Bruno Meinecke, "Music and Medicine in Classical Antiquity," in *Music and Medicine*, eds. Dorothy M. Schullian and Max Schoen (New York: Henry Schuman, 1948, reprinted by Books for Libraries Press, Freeport, N.Y.), p. 57.
15. Alvin, *Music Therapy*, p. 39.
16. Meinecke, "Music and Medicine in Classical Antiquity," p. 53.
17. Ibid.
18. Alvin, *Music Therapy*, p. 42.
19. H. E. Sigerist, *Civilization and Disease* (Chicago: University of Chicago Press, 1962, Phoenix Books edition), p. 133.

20. Alvin, *Music Therapy*, p. 42.
21. Sorell, *The Dance Through the Ages*, p. 27.
22. Herbert J. Muller, *The Loom of History* (New York: The New American Library of World Literature, Mentor Books, 1958), p. 450.
23. Ibid., pp. 113, 154.
24. Kenneth Clark, *Civilisation* (New York: Harper & Row, 1969), p. 50.
25. Sorell, *The Dance Through the Ages*, pp. 38–39.
26. Alvin, *Music Therapy*, p. 35.
27. H. E. Sigerist, "The Story of Tarantism," in Schullian and Schoen, *Music and Medicine;* Sorell, *The Dance Through the Ages;* G. M. Gould and Walter L. Pyle, *Anomalies and Curiosities of Medicine* (New York: The Julian Press, 1956).
28. Sigerist, "The Story of Tarantism," p. 114.
29. Alvin, *Music Therapy;* Sorell, *The Dance Through the Ages;* Sigerist, "The Story of Tarantism."
30. Quoted in Alvin, *Music Therapy*, pp. 96–97.
31. Alvin, *Music Therapy*, p. 98.
32. Ibid., p. 99.
33. Charles W. Hughes, "Rhythm and Health," in Schullian and Schoen, *Music and Medicine*, p. 175.
34. Vera Moretti, book review of Werner F. Kuemmel, *Music and Medicine as Interrelated in Theory and Practice from 800-1800*, in *Journal of Music Therapy* 15, no. 3 (Fall, 1978):158–59.
35. G. E. von Grunebaum, *Medieval Islam: A Study in Cultural Orientation* (Chicago: University of Chicago Press, 1954), p. 340.
36. Armen Carapetyan, "Music and Medicine in the Renaissance and in the 17th and 18th Centuries," in Schullian and Schoen, *Music and Medicine*, pp. 121–23.
37. Ibid., p. 124.
38. Ibid., p. 130.
39. Ibid.
40. Robert Burton, *The Anatomy of Melancholy*, Part 2, Sec. 2.
41. Alvin, *Music Therapy*, p. 47.
42. Carapetyan, "Music and Medicine in the Renaissance and in the 17th and 18th Centuries," p. 146.
43. Ibid., p. 148.
44. Gerald Carson, "The Victorians Revisited," in *The Human Side of History*, ed. R. F. Locke (New York: Hawthorn Books, 1970), pp. 34–35.
45. George Leonard, "The Rediscovery of the Body," *New York Magazine*, December 27, 1976/January 3, 1977, p. 39.
46. Bruce Haley, *The Healthy Body and Victorian Culture* (Cambridge, Mass.: Harvard University Press, 1978).

2

The Psychotherapeutic Bases

As we saw in the preceding chapter, the use of the expressive arts in therapy through the centuries was based on the intuitive recognition that the same wellsprings feed the streams of creativity and analysis, of thought and affect, of reflection and expression, of emotional state and physical condition.

During most of the history of the Western world, however, mind and body were separate — and distinctly unequal. Thinking was, if not supernatural, at least anatural in origin, in the sense that thought was unpredictable; it did not seem to follow the laws of nature that governed human physiology or the growth of plants or the movements of the planets. During the Age of Reason, the name the intellectuals of the time bestowed on the eighteenth century, a number of philosophers sought once again — as had the ancient Greeks — the universal laws of nature. Several questioned the traditional distinction between mind and body; Hobbes and Locke, for example, argued persuasively that the only world we can know is the one we experience through our senses, that our thinking is limited by our sensations, and that thought is not exempt from the laws of nature that govern the rest of the universe. By and large, however, until late in the nineteenth century, attempts to explain, predict, or control thought were conceived in mystical, rather than rational, terms.

PSYCHOLOGY AS THE SCIENCE OF MIND

The father of scientific psychology is generally considered to be Wilhelm Wundt, who in 1874 argued in his book, *Principles of Physiological Psychology*, that the mind must be subjected to the same objective and scientifically rigorous study that had been applied to the body since the Renaissance and the Scientific Revolution that followed. While Wundt was given permission to establish the first psychological laboratory at the University of Leipzig in 1879, the move suggested that the university administrators were indulging the whim of a professor, rather than encouraging a serious study of mind. Students who attended Wundt's lectures were granted no academic credit. Hence, the initial response to Wundt's innovation was less than overwhelming: four students came to his first lecture.

Wundt's basic thesis was that thinking, like blood circulation or muscle function, is a natural phenomenon that is subject to laws of nature and is therefore a suitable subject for rigorous scientific study. Had Wundt presented this position several decades earlier, he might well have been subjected to bitter attack from the clergy and from his own colleagues. Wundt, however, was fortunate in that just about this time a bitter controversy was raging over Darwin's startling contention that man himself was descended from lower forms of animal. Compared with Darwin's theory, Wundt's postulate was tame stuff, and it passed virtually unnoticed in the academic community.

By the mid-1880s, however, Wundt's psychological laboratory was attracting increasing numbers of students. The measurement processes that Wundt introduced were crude by today's standards, but they did take psychology out of the area of abstract philosophical conjecture into the sciences, where empirical data, rather than logic, constitute compelling evidence.

Out of the Leipzig laboratory came the disciples who were to carry to universities throughout the Western world the new gospel. Edward Bradford Titchener, one of Wundt's early students, became a professor of psychology at Cornell University, where he organized the new thinking about thinking into a theoretical system. To Titchener, psychology was the science of consciousness, "physics with the observer kept in." As in the other sciences, its findings are based on experience, which Titchener defined for psychology in terms of three components: sensations, such as hearing, touching, or seeing; affect or feelings; and images, such as dreams or memories. This approach to psychology, called *structuralism* because of its focus on basic units of experience, created almost immediately a number of challenges.

William James, the first native-born American psychologist, had studied physiology, anatomy, biology, and medicine at Harvard. He dropped out of school in a state of depression, but returned to obtain a medical degree in 1869. In 1872, he accepted an offer to teach physiology at Harvard, but restless and still depressed, he read widely in philosophy, seeking answers to explain his depression. By 1875, about the time that Wundt published his *Principles of Physiological Psychology*, James began to perceive a convergence between physiology and philosophy. In that year, he started a class in psychology, actually predating Wundt's psychological laboratory in Leipzig. James later reported that the first lecture he had ever heard on psychology was his own.

Like Wundt, James saw the new subject as a science, and he began psychological experiments. However, James's thinking led him to question the principles of structuralism, and his 1890 textbook, *The Principles of Psychology*, rejected the atomistic approach of Wundt and Titchener. James argued that the notion of isolated sensations divorced from accompanying associations is a fiction based on faulty analysis; it simply does not exist in the human mind. Thought, to James, involved a constant interaction of associations and revisions of experiences, sensations, and images in a constant flow.

To James, the heart of psychological investigation was the search for *function* rather than structure. Mental associations, he argued, help us not only to recognize an object for what it is, but define what it is in terms of function; mental associations help us to perform the appropriate tasks involved in dealing with an object. We not only recognize stairs, but prepare to climb them without having to analyze the steps or sequences involved. James believed that the focus on function helps to explain the process of turning tasks into habits; the more often we perform a task, such as walking or opening a door, the more likely it is that we will perform it automatically, without thinking about it.

From a summary discussion of three of the pioneers in psychology, it becomes clear that the early investigators were concerned more with the *study* of human thought and behavior than with its control, although some — like John B. Watson, the father of behaviorism — undertook to provide advice on such subjects as child rearing.

While the thrust of the early psychologists was to make the study of mind a science, it must be noted that processes of investigation in the field are considerably "softer" than in the physical or natural sciences. Both findings and conclusions tend to be highly tentative in psychology, and both tend to be highly susceptible to bias in the direction of the researcher's expectations.

The heart and soul of "scientific method" is the experiment — a study in a controlled environment in which extraneous variables can be isolated or eliminated. Thus, in a laboratory situation, the researcher can repeat an experiment, changing only one variable at a time. But the kinds of experimentation that will provide conclusive answers to many of the most vexing problems of human behavior are simply not to be permitted in our society. As a result, psychological "experimentation" involving human beings is likely to involve considerably less than complete isolation of variables.

Because of the difficulties involved in human experimentation, two methods have become standard operating procedure in psychological research. The first is the substitution of animals for human beings. Obviously, this form of surrogate experimentation has serious limitations. Ostensibly, it would appear to be analogous to medical experiments that involve laboratory animals. But the effects of a drug in inducing cancer in rats are hardly the equivalent of inferring and predicting complex human responses from situations based on the pecking of pigeons for food or the racing of rats through a maze, except on the very lowest levels of behavior.

The basis of most psychological findings, therefore, has become the *statistical correlation*. This correlation is a connection of two or more factors that examines the likelihood of one factor occurring if another, or others, occur. For example, it has often been noted that persons with high IQs tend to have children with higher than average IQs. As you may have perceived, this kind of simple correlation can stimulate more questions than answers. For unlike the case in the laboratory experiment, in which the variables can be isolated one at a time, the problem in identifying the reason for the correlation is formidable. It is possible that high IQ is inherited — and many psychologists subscribe to this hypothesis. But it is also possible that high-IQ parents create environments in which children *learn* to become high-IQ individuals — and many psychologists subscribe to *this* hypothesis. After several decades of investigation, and scores of ingenious research projects, the nature-versus-nurture debate still rages.

The methodology involved in finding statistical correlations rarely lends itself to the formulation of firm and unqualified conclusions. For one thing, even when a clear correlation can be identified, cause-and-effect relationships may not be at all clear. Moreover, the notion of correlation is based on the concept of *more likely*, rather than *either-or*. And the probabilities themselves are often less convincing than investigators may suggest or the layman would like to believe. They rest on what psychologists refer to as *statistical significance*. But words in statistics do not mean what they mean in everyday conversation. Significant, for example, does not mean *important*, or *major*, or *meaningful*, as it would in most communication; it simply means that the correlation is greater than would be expected on the basis of chance alone. In many cases, the relationships are significantly less than the term significant would suggest in normal discussion. One result is the production of sharply conflicting conclusions by psychological researchers and the painfully slow accretion of firmly grounded conclusions that are generally acceptable to psychologists.

But by far the most vexing problem in psychological research is a philosophical one. We are often not sure that the factor, or quality, or trait, being investigated even exists! Most of the subjects of investigation in psychology are *hypothetical constructs*. They are concepts, like *the unconscious*, that cannot be observed or measured directly, but are inferred and hypothesized from overt behavior. Such constructs are ways of explaining the world in which we live. They are inferences built up through the intersections and overlappings of many observations. They are not facts; they are attempts to explain facts. They may be adequate, reasonable, and satisfactory explanations, to the degree that they help us to understand, to predict, and to control the world. It should be remembered that until technology helped scientists establish their existence, *atoms* and *genes* were hypothetical constructs. History, on the other hand, is littered with the remains of such constructs that have been abandoned because they did not hold up over time as adequate explanations or predictors — constructs such as that of body humors, about which you read in the first chapter.

Because such constructs are not facts, they invite debate. The evidence on which their existence is predicated is often ambiguous and open to conflicting interpretations. For example, some psychoanalysts think that the phenomenon of posthypnotic suggestion is evidence that an unconscious exists. When an individual in his waking state obeys a suggestion that he had been given during hypnosis, they claim, the action is proof that the suggestion had been stored in his unconscious. On the other hand, the behaviorist Pavlov explained posthypnotic suggestion in terms of stimuli that had acted on subcortical areas of the brain during states of decreased alertness and diffusion of cortex inhibition. Behaviorists today point out that similar phenomena can be induced by the use of drugs, and they argue a neurochemical explanation.

It is readily apparent that in a field in which so much divergence of opinion exists, there is a wide range of "scientific" philosophy and methodology. At one end of the debate over consciousness, most humanists assert that the truly significant elements of consciousness are beyond direct observation. At the other end stands the assertion by John B. Watson, the father of modern behaviorism, that the whole notion of consciousness is a superstitious remnant of medieval thought and that the only fit subject for scientific investigation is the overt behavior that can be observed and measured. As we shall see, the divergence of views on the nature of the human psyche — in fact, on the very existence of a psyche — has profoundly influenced the methodologies in the various psychotherapies.

PSYCHOTHERAPY AS
APPLIED PSYCHOLOGY

The science of psychology, like science in general, may be viewed as an attempt to *understand*, to *predict*, and to *control* its subject. The obvious application of findings in psychology should be in the psychotherapies, and the outsider generally assumes that the therapies are built upon a solid research base of findings from experimental psychology. Indeed, some of the psychotherapies bear the names of psychologies, such as *gestalt* or *behaviorism*. In many cases, however, the approaches in psychotherapy bear only a tenuous relationship to theoretical formulations or research in the parent psychology.

The major reason for the divergence of psychology and psychotherapy is that it is far easier to identify general laws of behavior, as Wundt did in his Leipzig laboratory, than it is to account for individual differences. The psychological theories built on such generalizations are, therefore, more helpful in explaining or even predicting the behavior of large groups of people than in predicting the behavior of an individual. Thus, to the degree that psychotherapy deals with individual differences, it can make only limited use of psychological research findings. By and large, psychotherapists were already practicing therapy when they formulated their theories of personality. The theories came out of the practice, out of clinical observations, rather than out of the kind of research that is demanded by most experimental psychologists.

As a result of the different views of what constitutes adequate research, psychotherapy itself is perhaps more controversial a subject within the field of psychology than it is among the general public. Many academic or research psychologists (the "hard-headed" or "tough-minded" psychologists, as they term themselves) tend to look with disdain on the clinicians (the "soft-headed" or "tender-minded" psychologists) who practice, in the view of the researchers, a fuzzy and undefined art that smacks of mysticism. It is painfully true that it is extremely difficult to measure the effectiveness of one form of psychotherapy against another or even to document a correlation between treatment and cure. Outcome studies in psychotherapy that raise questions about the effectiveness of various therapies, or of therapy in general, have stimulated a bitter debate within the profession itself that centers on the question of whether psychotherapy is a science, an art, or a form of faith healing.

Hans J. Eysenck, a psychologist at the University of London's Institute of Psychiatry, produced a number of studies some years ago that focused on the efficacy of psychotherapy. Among his conclusions: neurotic disorders tend to be self-limiting, psychoanalysis is no more successful than any other method, and — for neurotics, at any rate — "all methods of psychotherapy fail to improve on the recovery rate obtained through ordinary life-experiences and nonspecific treatment."[1]

Since the publication of Eysenck's views, other studies have been conducted; some reinforce Eysenck's conclusions, while others dispute them. What is most significant about Eysenck's work is the furor it created in the psychotherapeutic community and the defensiveness that surfaced. The very act of testing the effectiveness of psychotherapy, he reported, aroused emotional opposition that he found analogous to that of a true believer against a blasphemer who had attempted a statistical test of the efficiency of prayer.[2]

Fortunately, the kind of defensiveness into which Eysenck ran is waning. As a result of several decades of investigation on the outcome of psychotherapy, all but the most faithful have come to accept the need for more than the uncorroborated anecdotal reports of cures that, to many of the newer breed of psychotherapy researchers, are reminiscent of mystical miracle cures. As a result, the controlled study has increasingly come to represent the standard method of evaluation in the field of psychotherapy.

The controlled study, unlike the anecdotal reports that still swell the pages of the professional journals, involves the use of both an experimental group and a control group; the latter group may receive a placebo, like a sugar pill, or no treatment at all, so that a basis exists for comparison. The most refined form of controlled study involves what is known as a *double-blind* approach, in which neither the patient nor the therapist knows which is the experimental group and which is the control group. An increasing number of investigators have begun to apply in psychotherapy the kind of measurement and evaluation techniques that have long been used in the sciences.

Psychotherapy, whether or not it is a science, does represent the Establishment in the field of mental health, and its practitioners have, in the words of Martin Gross, become "the new seers" of Western society. "By offering us the *hidden truth* behind virtually every act of our waking hours," he writes in his book, *The Psychological Society*, psychotherapists have "seized the role society once divided among the clergy, philosophers and statesmen — and in earlier times among the oracles, prophets, even magicians."[3]

Despite the recognition among many research psychologists of the interrelatedness of mind and body, the profession adheres, by and large, to the technique of "the talking cure," and practitioners tend to look down on any but verbal therapies. However, the growing research element in psychotherapy may, in time, turn the field upside down. A suspicion is growing among some researchers that the most effective approaches in therapy may include some that had once been considered supportive or adjunctive.

The leadership in the fields of mental health and human behavior, however, still consists of largely verbal psychotherapists. The prevailing theories and techniques of the various schools of psychotherapy are often contradictory, but they exert a profound influence on the emerging nonverbal therapies.

Psychoanalysis: The Hidden Wellsprings of Behavior

Despite the increasing popularization of a host of newer, and frequently more dramatic, therapies, the bulk of practitioners in the field still adhere to the psychoanalytic school. One 1970 study revealed that two-thirds of the psychiatrists surveyed called themselves "Freudian," and the majority of psychotherapists used techniques derived from the theories of Sigmund Freud or his disciples.[4] In addition to psychiatrists (who hold M.D. degrees), a host of Ph.D. psychologists and clinical (also called psychiatric) social workers, with M.S.W. degrees, practice a variety of therapies, most of which can be described as Freudian or neo-Freudian.

Psychoanalysis is largely the invention of Sigmund Freud who, unlike Wundt or James, was a practicing physician, a neurologist, rather than a scientist or an academician. His theories evolved from his medical practice and were largely intuitively derived; they also established the medical model, which is the standard in the field of mental health (the term itself is drawn from medicine). Freud himself was willing to make use of the analytical methods of other disciplines, and he even proposed training such professionals as teachers and clergymen in the practical application of psychoanalytic methods.[5] However, when the American Psychoanalytic Association was founded, its members declared themselves opposed to the training of nonmedical professionals and to membership in the organization of any but physicians. Membership subsequently was opened to others, but the narrow medical base was early established for psychoanalysis.

Freud's ideas were at variance with those of his American counterparts. Although Freud visited the United States in 1909 (James attended one of his lectures), it was not until the 1920s that his approach began to find favor in this country; since that time, it has been the basis for most of the psychotherapy done by American psychiatrists.

Freud believed that much of our behavior is based on hidden motives and unconscious wishes. The psyche is constantly engaged in internal battles in which childish wishes and "instinctual demands" are repressed and forced out of consciousness, only to surface in dreams and fantasies or in "Freudian slips" — the absentminded mistakes that reveal underlying preoccupations. Psychoanalysis is based on the assumption that the problems that plague adults have their origins in early childhood, during which the child represses painful sensations, perceptions, and feelings. Adult fears correspond with early childish wishes that the individual had censored, and repressed emotions are related to aggressive or sexual drives that the child perceived as dangerous. In large part, contended Freud, this repression is an attempt by the child to deny impulses or desires that are frowned upon by the controlling adults. These repressed wishes and urges survive, seething in the realm of the unconscious, from which they emerge in uncontrollable ways. Psychoanalysis is seen as a method by which these repressed feelings and wishes are brought into consciousness, largely through *free association* of seemingly unrelated ideas and thoughts that provide clues to the underlying problems, or through *dream interpretation.* Once at the conscious level, the repressed feelings and impulses can be recognized and dealt with rationally — with the help, of course, of a trained analyst.

At the heart of Freudian psychoanalysis are a number of concepts that are interrelated into a coherent structure. The essential elements of the Freudian system are a series of constructs and postulates: that the human psyche consists of *conscious, preconscious,* and *unconscious* levels of awareness; that primary thought processes originate in the unconscious level and have their own independent energies and images; that the secondary process involves conscious awareness, logical thinking, and deliberate (as opposed to unconscious) symbol formation; and that the *ego* acts as a mediator between these often opposing and conflicting forces.

Central to the Freudian system is the division of the personality into *id, ego,* and *superego.* To Freud, the *id* is the oldest of the mental provinces; it includes the basic human instincts and drives with which an individual is born. Freud called the id "the obscure inaccessible part of our personality." He wrote in his *New Introductory Lectures on Psychoanalysis:*

> We can come nearest to the id with images, and call it a chaos, a cauldron of seething excitement. We suppose that it is somewhere in direct contact with somatic processes, and takes over from them instinctual needs and gives them mental expression. . . . The laws of logic — above all, the law of contradiction — do not hold for processes of the id. . . . Naturally, the id knows no values, no good and evil, no morality. . . . Instinctual cathexes seeking discharge — that, in our view, is all that the id contains.[6]

The id has no direct contact with the outside world. It is the constant infant, demanding the instant gratification of desires. The major way in which the id communicates with the conscious is through dreams, which are the externalization of internal processes, and through those odd mistakes known as "Freudian slips."

The *ego* is the "I" — the agency that mediates between the inner and outer worlds. From the outside world, it gathers information through the senses. It has the task of self-preservation, and, to this end, it controls the processes of thinking and reasoning. In contrast with the id, which operates on the "pleasure principle," the ego is governed by the "reality principle." Thus, it protects the individual against the unreasonable demands of the id, which seeks nothing more than the indiscriminate satisfaction of its cravings. The ego, then, controls the id by channeling its energies into realistic actions; the ego may, therefore, postpone or suppress the demands of the id.

The combination of ego and id alone would constitute an effective psychic organism if individuals lived in isolation. Since individuals live in society with other individuals, however, adult behavior is conditioned by morality as well as by effectiveness. So Freud postulated a moral guardian that he called the *superego* that internalizes the inhibiting forces of the outside world — the judgments and standards of the adults who control the behavior of the child. The superego eventually becomes the successor of the parents and teachers who indoctrinate the young child during the formative years; it is the institutionalization and internalization of what is commonly called "conscience," and it monitors and censors. Whereas the *ego* controls behavior in the direction of effectiveness and survival, the *superego* directs it into socially acceptable channels.

Successful therapy, in Freudian analytic practice, depends on "authentic" communication by the patient — that is, a free and uninhibited release of repressed feelings and urges. The primary vehicle for such release is *free association,* or the exposure of internal associations of apparently unrelated thoughts and words; these associations provide clues to repressions that are struggling for expression. Analysis, furthermore, requires neutrality on the part of the analyst, who must be careful not to "cue" the patient or to force a response in a way that would interfere with authentic expression.

It is this area of authentic expression, in particular, that holds promise for the expressive arts therapies in the Freudian model. The mechanism for the interrelationship between the conscious and the unconscious, to Freud, was the level of images just below the level of awareness; this level Freud identified as the *preconscious.* In order to deal with the preconscious, it is necessary to accept the irrational, and the communication between the conscious and the unconscious is expressed symbolically through images. This expression of the primary forces was explored by Freud in his monumental *The Inter-*

pretation of Dreams, in which he identified dreams as revelations of internal processes that focus on the demands of the unconscious.

The functioning of the preconscious level is of particular interest in the arts therapies, where spontaneity as *authentic self-expression* coincides with spontaneity as *creative production*. In psychoanalysis, dream interpretation and free association are the major tools for the exploration of the unconscious. To many in the expressive arts therapies, the actual creative expression of the unconscious through works of art, music, or movement makes overt what would otherwise be covert operations. As we shall see in later chapters, they are frequently less susceptible to inhibiting influences than are verbal expressions. Freud pointed out that "all of our dreams are preponderantly visual,"[7] an observation that lays much of the basis for the frequently applied expression in visual arts therapy that patients' works are frozen fragments of dreams that have been exposed and preserved for examination.

While Freud's work remains the basis of much of the psychotherapy practiced in this country (this is not true in much of Europe; British psychiatrists tend to be behavioristically oriented), some major problems exist in the application of traditional Freudian psychoanalysis to certain groups of patients. As Freud himself pointed out, the effectiveness of analysis depends largely on the motivation of the patient to deal rationally with his unconscious feelings as they surface. Psychoanalysis, therefore, is better suited for *neurotics** than for *psychotics* — those whose behavior is characterized by severely disordered thought and inappropriate emotions and reactions.

Freud's theoretical formulations have been the center of debate from the beginning; in fact, some of his most brilliant disciples and colleagues broke with him on points of theory or practice. Indeed, it is almost remarkable to note the propensity of Freud's associates to create divergent theories. This phenomenon has its roots in the fact that, for all its brilliance as a comprehensive theory, the Freud-

---

*The term "neurosis" was used by Freud to describe the result of the battle between the ego and the id. Because it is vague enough to describe essentially well individuals, the American Psychiatric Association's 1980 edition of the *Diagnostic and Statistical Manual of Mental Disorders* substituted the term "anxiety disorders." The change provoked objections from large numbers of psychoanalysts who saw the move as a repudiation of Freud's theory of personality. Despite the official abandonment of the term, "neurosis" is likely to persist in the literature and conversation of psychoanalysis for some time.

ian concept of personality was built from personal observation and personal experience rather than a solid body of research findings. The bulk of personality theory — Freudian and non-Freudian alike — has been built on the basis of clinical observation, a method that makes personality theory highly susceptible to the biases of the theorist and to the influences of the environment in which he or she practices. Given the method, it is not surprising that many of Freud's concepts were highly personal projections, colored by his personality, his own childhood experiences, the composition of his clientele, and the nature of Viennese society at the turn of the century.

Many of Freud's critics charge that he projected his own biases and idiosyncracies into universal stages of development and norms of behavior. Freud's one-time associate Carl Jung asserted that from the day of their first meeting in 1907, Jung realized that sexuality had for Freud an emotional commitment that made it a central principle with the quality nearly of a religion.[8] Moreover, Freud's theories were developed in the context of a social climate that no longer exists, a fact that leads many modern therapists — including psychoanalysts — to consider much of classical Freudian theory outdated in specifics, if not in concept. Freud's middle-class and upper-class patients were stifled by the bonds of the prevailing social and moral codes. Many psychotherapists argue that a more prevalent problem today is the search for guidelines to behavior, rather than the need to escape them.

Nevertheless, it must be remembered that Freudian theory laid the foundation for modern psychotherapy. On the one hand, it invited outrageous oversimplifications and popularizations, as during the 1920s when psychoanalysis was touted as a panacea for all mental problems, in which cures would begin simultaneously with free expression and with the identification of the patient's disorder. On the other hand, it served as a basis for refinements in theory building — an invitation that was seized eagerly by many of Freud's own disciples and associates. While those of Freud's colleagues who broke with the master tended to retain the central features of his theory — the concept of the unconscious, for example — some of them reshaped their theories in ways that have tended to make them particularly attractive to many practitioners in the expressive arts therapies.

Carl Gustave Jung had been an associate of Freud in Vienna, but a number of basic theoretical disagreements persuaded him to leave Freud's circle in 1913 to establish a therapy of his own, known as *analytical psychotherapy*. While much of Jung's thinking builds on Freud's ideas, his overwhelming contribution to psychological theory is his expansion and development of the idea of the unconscious. Unlike Freud's depository of repressed desires — "a cauldron of seething excitations" — Jung's unconscious was a rich, wide source of ideas and symbols from which the ego draws strength and vitality.

Jungian therapy is largely devoted to facilitating the dialogue between the conscious and the unconscious. The dialogue is a two-way communication, and it is conducted largely through the media of dreams and symbols. A word or image, wrote Jung, "is symbolic when it implies more than its obvious and immediate meaning. It has a wider 'unconscious' aspect that is never precisely defined or fully explained. . . . As the mind explores the symbol, it is led to ideas that lie beyond the grasp of reason."[9]

Unconscious aspects of our perception of reality exist, according to Jung, that include the translation of sensed phenomena into perceptions, a process he calls *psychic events*. The unconscious, believed Jung, is a friend and an advisor and provides signs and symbols for our guidance. "It is a basic tenet of Jungian therapy," wrote E. C. Whitmont and Yoram Kaufmann, "that all products of the unconscious are symbolic and can be taken as guiding messages. Thus, the symptoms, the neurosis itself, are not merely indications of psychic malfunctioning, but show the way out of the conflict underlying them, if symbolically understood."[10]

Jung's concern with the symbolic messages from the unconscious led to the development of a number of concepts that have served as the basis for many of the techniques in the expressive arts therapies. In particular, he postulated two levels of the unconscious. The *personal unconscious* contains those experiences that have been unnoticed, forgotten, or repressed — the myriad of phenomena that have been pushed out of the conscious mind or that, as Jung put it, are not yet "ripe for consciousness." Here, they are organized into *complexes*, or collections of associated concepts and images in an emotional context that color an individual's thoughts and behavior.

It is the complex — the cluster of experiences and associations — and not a single association that reveals, through free association, those areas that Jung called "the tender spots of the psyche, which react most quickly to an external stimulus or disturbance." Because such feelings and concepts are tied into a network, he concluded, free association can lead to "the critical secret thoughts."[11]

Jung's most original and untraditional formulation was that of a deeper level of the unconscious, one of primordial imagery that is common to all humans. This collective unconscious is a storehouse of the accumulated memories and influences that have been inherited from past generations. Jung wrote:

> This psychic life is the mind of our ancient ancestors, the way in which they thought and felt, the way in which they conceived of life and the world, of gods and human beings. The existence of these historical layers is presumably the source of the belief in reincarnation and in memories of past lives. . . . There is no reason for believing that the psyche, with its peculiar structure, is the only thing in the world that has no history beyond its individual manifestation. Even the conscious mind cannot be denied a history extending over at least five thousand years. It is only individual ego-consciousness that has forever a new beginning and an early end. But the unconscious psyche is not only immensely old, it is also able to grow increasingly into an equally remote future. It forms, and is part of, the human species just as much as the body, which is also individually ephemeral, yet collectively of immeasurable duration.[12]

Jung pointed to the evolutionary sequence of our anatomy that is recapitulated from conception to birth. As the fetus grows within the womb, it resembles other species and even develops during the gestation period such specific features as gill slits and a tail. He thought it strange indeed to assume that the evolutionary sequence of experience cannot be recapitulated in the individual human and retained as unconscious memories that are common to all humanity. The collective concepts themselves Jung designated *archetypes,* universal concepts that are expressed in metaphors.

What themes, Jung asked, are repeated in art and literature, folklore and mythology, religion and philosophy? Why does virtually every culture tell stories that are remarkably similar — stories of divine beings who come to earth to mingle with the inhabitants, for example? Why does the theme of the angry mother recur in tales about wicked witches, cruel stepmothers, and she-devils? To Jung, these are manifestations of shared racial memories. He believed that humans can benefit from developing an increased awareness of the accumulated wisdom stored in their collective unconscious, and much of his therapy was focused on facilitating this awareness. To Jung, a basic function of consciousness is to heed the unconscious, which is not only the accumulation of a lifetime of repressions, but the wellspring of creativity and the source of guidance.

Obviously, then, Jungian psychology is a rich source of significant ideas for both psychological understanding and the creative process, a duality that makes Jung's ideas particularly attractive to the expressive arts therapies. In particular, the Jungian concern with the manifestations of the archetypes has laid the groundwork for much work done in visual arts therapy. The archetypal images, such as transformation, death and rebirth, the hero struggle, the father-god, the great mother and the divine child, are expressed differently within each culture, but they are persistent and prevalent.

Both the manifestations of the collective unconscious and the expressions of the personal unconscious eventually were focused in Jungian *mandalas*, circular symbolic drawings that Jung considered cryptograms. To Jung, the circle itself is an archetypal symbol of unity, and he noted that throughout history, the circular mandala reappears in a variety of forms, from the sand drawings of primitive peoples to the round, stained-glass windows of Gothic cathedrals. But while the forms vary from culture to culture, the mandala itself represents a constant and recurring form.

Jung's discovery of the mandala (perhaps rediscovery would be more appropriate, since he was not the first to note the significance of the circle or of circular drawings) was, significantly, in the form of a personal artistic expression; in a sense, it provides a key to his entire system. He wrote that when he began drawing mandalas, he found that "it became increasingly plain to me that the mandala is the center. It is the exponent of all paths. It is the path to the center, to individuation."[13]

Because of Jung's regard for imagination and for creativity as healing forces, Jungian psychotherapy, even more than Freudian psychoanalysis, constitutes a rich source of approaches for the practitioner in the expressive arts therapies. Jung's emphasis on active imagination techniques, in contrast with Freud's rather passive use of free association, encourages the patient to fantasize and to explore. Feelings are examined and explored through a variety of approaches — in painting, sculpture, music, and movement. And Jung's concept of the collective unconscious, the psychic heritage of mankind, is fundamentally a communication of *images* from generation to generation. It is in the search for the common language of imagery, unencumbered by cultural dialect and geographic determinism, that arts therapists find Jungian therapy so attractive. The projection and development of images through nonverbal means creates for the arts therapist a treasury of diagnostic and therapeutic instruments. Moreover, Jung's "individuation" is creative and imaginative; it converges with artistic creativity.

Jungian therapists often argue that Jung's theories are built on a more solid empirical base than Freud's. Jung explored widely in other disciplines and drew from an enormous body of information in the arts, the humanities, and the sciences. (Jung's first argument with Freud, in 1908, was the result of Jung's conjecture that *dementia praecox*, now called schizophrenia, has an organic cause — a toxin that attacks the brain. The chemical basis of psychosis is currently receiving a good deal of attention and considerable experimental support.) At bottom, however, his theory, like Freud's, reflects the biases, interests, and predispositions of its creator. Jung's concern with the mysterious and the mystical, reflected in his theory of personality and in such concepts as that of "synchronicity" — an acausal principle that connects seemingly unrelated events — is no more susceptible to testing than Freud's hypothetical constructs.

Because it has been viewed as highly mystical, Jungian psychotherapy has been dormant in this country, and its practitioners relatively few. However, it appears to be gaining in popularity due, perhaps, to the rediscovery of Jung by arts therapists to whom his theories are particularly attractive (and perhaps to the rising interest in the mystical and the occult). The number of applicants for the C. G. Jung Foundation's training institute in New York has been growing in recent years.

Along with Jung, the other outstanding leader of the palace revolt against Freud was Alfred Adler, who actually broke from Freud's discussion group, the Psychological Wednesday Society, two years earlier than Jung. Adler had been one of the Viennese analysts who had objected to Freud's "anointment" of the Swiss foreigner Jung as his crown prince or heir apparent (the terms are Freud's). This revolt was not the cause of Adler's defection, which, like Jung's, was based on disagreements over theory.

Like Jung, Adler objected to Freud's emphasis on sexuality, especially his stress on infant sexuality. Adler agreed with Freud that human behavior is conditioned by unconscious inborn drives, but for Adler, the dominant urges are social in nature. Humans, to Adler, are creatures of social forces to which they must adjust throughout their lives. Most of Adler's terms have meaning only in a social context: "inferiority complex," the attempt to overcome feelings of inferiority; "masculine protest," the (culturally influenced) masculine drive toward power as one way of dealing with a sense of inferiority; "lifestyle."

Adler believed that human development in a social environment inevitably creates feelings of inferiority. The helpless infant, dependent for very life on the adults in the environment, is constantly reminded of his or her inferior status. Parents and teachers are constantly pointing out children's faults and correcting them. To compensate for the resultant sense of inferiority, most individuals set goals of achievement for themselves that will give them either a sense of mastery and superiority or a sense of personal fulfillment. The specific goals may be realistic or unrealistic. They may be healthy or they may be neurotic, as in the case of an individual who uses illness or helplessness as a means of controlling others. The fundamental goal on which an individual focuses then becomes the dominant thrust of that individual's life.

An understanding of any person, therefore, requires an understanding of his or her cognitive organization, the *lifestyle*, or set of principles that helps that person understand, predict, and control experience. This lifestyle represents the filters through which any individual sees experience—and all of life. Phenomenology or subjectivity, therefore, is the key to understanding an individual. "We must be able to see with his eyes," Adler wrote, "and listen with his ears."[14] While behavior may change, a lifestyle remains fairly constant throughout a person's life, unless it is changed through the intervention of psychotherapy.

Adler's emphasis, unlike Freud's, was on the conscious, and particularly on the role of the ego in shaping personality. To Adler, humans are not creatures of instinctual urges and unconscious drives that must constantly be battled; they have the freedom to choose alternative responses to problems, although these choices may be influenced by crystallized lifestyles and apperceptive biases. During the developing years, particularly, individuals are free to choose their own destinies and help shape their own lifestyles. As opposed to Freudian reductionism (the notion that individuals are composed of distinct and antagonistic parts), Adlerian psychology sees humans as holistic and indivisible, creative, responsible, and "becoming," rather than "being." If these terms have an oddly modern ring, it should be noted that Adler is frequently viewed as a precursor of the humanist psychotherapies that abound on the current scene. In fact, Albert Ellis calls Adler "one of the first humanistic psychologists."[15]

Adler also discounted Freud's medical model, seeing the psychopath as "discouraged," rather than "sick." He rejected both psychomatic and somatopsychic hypotheses, insisting that the key question is not whether the mind affects the body or the body affects the mind, but how the whole self is involved in the pursuit of goals, a view that has significant meaning for movement therapy in particular and that presaged the development of many of the newer psychotherapies.

Many of Adler's ideas have found their way into two groups of therapy: transactional analysis and the humanistic therapies. It is through the latter group, especially, that Adlerian psychotherapy has had its major influence on the arts therapies.

It is interesting that despite their general influence on psychotherapeutic theory, neither Jung nor Adler has significantly influenced the mainstream of psychoanalytic practice in this country. This absence of impact may be due in large part to the domination of psychoanalysis by Freud himself during his lifetime. Since Freud's death in 1939, however, there have been widespread and rapid changes in psychoanalytic theory and practice, notably: a deemphasis on sexuality as the central factor in personality development, a growing interest in environmental factors in the shaping of personality, the exploration of the superego in terms of comparative value systems, and a growing concern with the issue of interpersonal relationships. In connection with this last subject, two names demand at least passing mention.

Harry Stack Sullivan was an American psychiatrist who, like the others we have discussed, moved from a Freudian view of personality to one of his own. He carried Adler's interest in social relationships further out of the individual psyche into the arena of social interaction. He stressed the "observable interactions between and among people, rather than the hypothesized inner workings of the psyche," writes Donn Byrne of Purdue University. "In fact, he identified psychiatry with social psychology and recognized that personality is an abstract construct derived from observed social interactions."[16]

Sullivan was essentially an environmentalist whose approach assumed that personality development is a dynamic process and that change is possible. Interpersonal relationships during the first few years are limited almost entirely to the family, and it is in this context that personality traits are developed. By the time the child goes to school, the superego is formed and the personality jells. Relations with other people depend largely on *transferences* from the early family structure and are heavily influenced by the mixture of gratifications and frustrations that the individual had experienced within the family. For Freud's pleasure principle as a major instinctual drive, Sullivan substituted a search for security that underlies much of interpersonal relations.

Sullivan's *self* consists of a trinity, described in quite modern terms that are easily understood by the nonprofessional and that are forerunners of terms in some of the current "games" theories of interpersonal relations, such as transactional analysis. It consists of a *good-me*, a *bad-me*, and a *not-me*. The good-me is the healthy (nonneurotic) self-image that flows from the security of warm family relationships. The bad-me is the negative image that results from contacts in a hostile or threatening environment. The not-me is the complex of dissociated feelings that result from traumas and that may surface from time to time during emotional crises; the not-me is rejected by the individual as a false image that is not recognizable.

The ideas of Karen Horney closely resemble some of Sullivan's. Horney, a German-born, British-trained psychoanalyst, rejected a number of basic Freudian principles to develop her own theory. Like Sullivan, Horney believed that human social relationships are heavily influenced by family relationships during the child's formative years. To Horney, as to Sullivan, the dominant drive is the search for security, and — depending on the nature of the family's interactions — the child will adopt one of three survival strategies: moving toward people (submission), moving away from people (detachment), and moving against people (aggression).

Horney has come to be known as a feminist theorist, in large part because of her rejection of many of Freud's ideas that she considered sexist. Horney recognized the influence of sex-role expectations and social discrimination based on sex in the formation of personality. For example, where Freud had theorized that a woman's emotional life was controlled by her childhood wish for a penis, Horney asserted that envy by women was focused on the social privileges that men enjoy, such as independence, work security, and sexual freedom, rather than on anatomy.

The proliferation of divergent, psychoanalytically based therapies has spurred an internecine warfare within the ranks of the American Psychoanalytic Association on such issues as training standards, theory, and practice. In contrast with the classical Freudian analysts, whom they sometimes deride as the "kosher" analysts, the neo-Freudians tend to deemphasize the use of the traditional couch and to shorten the length of treatment. In turn, many Freudians insist that others practice a "psychoanalytically oriented psychotherapy," rather than psychoanalysis. The conflict reached such intensity during the 1950s that Robert P. Knight, as outgoing president of the American Psychoanalytic Association, chided the membership:

> The spectacle of a national association of physicians and scientists feuding with each other . . . and calling each other orthodox and conservative or deviant and dissident is not an attractive one, to say the least. Such terms belong to religions, or to fanatical political movements, and not to science and medicine. Psychoanalysis should be neither a "doctrine" nor a "party line." Perhaps we are still standing too much in the shadow of that giant, Sigmund Freud, to permit ourselves to view psychoanalysis as a science of the mind rather than as the doctrine of a founder.[17]

Despite the internal bickerings among psychoanalysts, however, (which seem to have subsided considerably since the 1950s as analysts have come increasingly to adopt "eclectic" approaches), the agreements among the various schools of psychoanalysis have always outweighed the differences. Except for a few mavericks like Adler, the neo-Freudians accept two of Freud's basic assumptions: that the determinants of human personality may be found in the dynamics of the unconscious; and that mental problems, like physical problems, are symptoms of "illness."

The medical model assumes further that problematic or abnormal behavior itself is not treatable, since it is only a symptom of an underlying problem. Only dealing with the problem itself can lead to a cure. A change in the behavior alone, with no resolution of the problem, would simply lead to the substitution of another behavioral symptom. To psychoanalysts in general, the resolution of the problem itself involves recognition of the causes by tracing the problem to its origin, and then grappling with it on a cognitive, or thinking, level, as well as on an affective one. As we shall see, all of these ideas — *symptom substitution*, the need to find the source of the problem, and, indeed, the medical model itself — are viewed with considerable skepticism by the advocates of both behaviorism and humanism. The medical model, moreover, is the subject of a bitter debate among psychiatrists themselves.

Such "radical" psychiatrists as R. D. Laing, Thomas Szaz, and Thomas Scheff argue that the term mental illness is merely a device for identifying and stigmatizing nonconformists whose behavior deviates from social norms. Critics point to studies showing that psychiatrists who come before courts and parole boards to identify potentially dangerous individuals have an accuracy rate of just above

50 percent, slightly higher than the odds obtained by flipping a coin. Such prognostic inaccuracy, they argue, would be considered intolerable in any other branch of medicine.

In his controversial book, *The Death of Psychiatry*, E. Fuller Torrey sees the concept of mental illness as a device by which psychiatrists seek to monopolize their roles as secular priests in a sick society.[18] Their public advice, in the words of social historian Christopher Lasch, ranges from "childbearing to the psychic qualifications of Presidential candidates . . . [and encourages] the widespread inclination to regard all social and political problems as psychiatric problems."[19] Just as priests once defined good and evil for society, Lasch contends, psychiatrists now distinguish between mental sickness and health, reality, and illusion.[20]

Despite the attacks, the medical practitioners are still in control of the field, as is evidenced by the persistence of such terms as *mental health, mental illness* — and *therapy* itself. Part of the public faith in psychiatry is attributable to the prestige of physicians in our society and to a prevalent confidence that medical doctors can cope with problems that are labeled *illnesses.* No small part of the control by medical practitioners is due to the fact that only they, among psychotherapists, have the keys to the medicine cabinet; they are legally permitted to deal effectively with patients who are unresponsive to therapy by prescribing and dispensing drugs to pacify and control the more severely disordered of their disturbed clientele.

During the debate over the revision of the American Psychiatric Association's diagnostic manual in the late 1970s, nonmedical therapists rose in anger at the medical nature of many of the new definitions. "The advance intelligence on the *DSM-III* reportedly has it turning every human problem into a disease," wrote George Albee, a past president of the American Psychological Association, "in anticipation of the shower of health-plan gold that is over the horizon." Albee argues that most of the emotional problems of living are not diseases and that to attribute most life crises to biological defects or biochemical conditions "is to sell our psychological birthright for short-term gain."[21]

Before leaving the subject of psychoanalysis, it should be made clear that, contrary to popular impression, not all psychiatrists are psychoanalysts and that not all psychoanalysts are psychiatrists. A major change in psychoanalysis has been the opening of membership in the prestigious American Psychoanalytic Association to nonmedical practitioners. While such nonphysicians are still in a small minority, they include such prominent individuals as writer Erik Erikson and theoretician Anna Freud, the master's daughter.

Behavior Therapy: The Behavior Is the Problem

While behaviorism as a practical psychology is at least as old as reliance on reward and punishment to shape behavior, the birth of modern American behaviorism may be traced to John B. Watson, who rose to prominence in the 1920s. Watson not only believed in environmental influences on the development of the individual, but contended that children could be conditioned for genius or stupidity. He rejected any notion of the unconscious, or even of consciousness itself.

Watson was the first student to receive a doctorate in psychology from the University of Chicago, where he wrote a dissertation on learning in rats. At the time, Titchener's view of psychology as the science of consciousness was the conventional wisdom in the field, and Watson was asked to conjecture on the kinds of consciousness that would account for the behavior he had noted. Watson was skeptical that rats have any consciousness at all, but he complied with departmental demands in order to get his doctorate. He persisted, however, in questioning the existence of constructs that could be neither observed nor measured.

In 1913, Watson wrote an article, "Psychology as the Behaviorist Views It," in which he contended that the idea of consciousness, of a mental life independent of behavior, is a superstition.[22] The unconscious, argued Watson, like the concept of soul, is a notion for which there is no empirical evidence; neither can be defined, observed, or measured. Such concepts, he contended, are theological inventions to cover our ignorance about biological processes. There is no evidence, for example, that dreams are messages from the unconscious. They may very well be biologically induced responses to specific physical stimuli, or manifestations of changes in the neurological and biochemical circuitry of the body. Psychology, he insisted, should be the science, not of consciousness, but of behavior. It is not necessary to postulate such constructs as the id, personality traits, inferred motivations, or causes of disorders, in order to explain, predict, or control behavior. In fact, he argued, behavior can be modified more effectively by abandoning such concepts and dealing directly with the behavior itself.

Watson's thinking was influenced in large part by the work of Ivan Pavlov, a Russian neurologist who demonstrated that dogs can be "conditioned" to salivate, not only when they are given food, but when the stimuli associated with feeding are present. Pavlov hypothesized that all behavior is a response to stimuli and that stimuli can be associated to create desired responses. Watson's own experiments showed that behavior changes can be induced without any reference to consciousness or mentalism; learning, he insisted, is based less on reasoning than on response to one's environment.

The father of modern behaviorism was no more immune to the influences of his own environment than had been the founder of psychoanalysis. His personality quirks, his biases, and social conditions found expression in his theories of personality. Watson himself wrote in 1924 that the increasing urbanization of the 1920s, and the accompanying social changes, colored his view that "the starting point for psychology is the study . . . of our neighbor" rather than self-introspection. And a fellow student at the University of Chicago recalled that Watson always had difficulty in making the introspective reports that were part of the investigative technique of the day. "Some of us speculated in later years," the student is reported to have said, "as to whether this fact may not have supplied some of the urge which eventually drove him toward a purely behavioristic system."[23]

Behaviorism has changed since Watson's day, largely as the result of the work of a handful of outstanding researchers. To most Americans today, behaviorist theory is associated with the name of B. F. Skinner, a Harvard psychologist who has pioneered in the field of operant conditioning. Skinner rejected the Pavlovian stimulus-response sequence upon which Watson had built his classical conditioning approach, because he was interested only in what *reinforced* behavior, not in what *caused* it. Skinner also modified Watson's original manifesto to the point where he deals with both overt and covert activities, on the ground that thinking itself is simply behavior. The basic principles, though, have not changed. Behaviorism as a psychology is still based on laboratory-validated concepts, and research centers on attempts to develop empirically based generalizations about observable behavior.

As a therapy, behaviorism is more concerned with changing behavior than with seeking causes for "maladjustive" behavior. The growth of behavior therapy, or behavior modification, has been remarkable. It has been seized upon in schools as a pragmatic approach to the problem of handling disruptive behavior or of coaxing reluctant pupils to the troughs of learning, often using such stimuli as M&Ms and candy bars. It has also been used as the basis for coping with social and personal needs, which range from the desire to stop smoking to rehabilitation of criminal offenders.

Behaviorist researchers are fond of citing research findings that seem to discredit some of the assumptions underlying the psychiatric medical model: for example, the assertion that treating maladjustive behavior (the symptom) without treating the underlying "cause" will simply create the substitution of one symptom for another. These studies, they contend, simply do not support the claims that symptom substitution occurs, that such substitution can be predicted in advance, and that the development of new symptoms would necessarily support the psychoanalytic theory.[24]

Behaviorists reject inferences about causes; they argue that references to needs, motives, impulses, and drives are unnecessary in predicting or controlling behavior. A central thesis underlying behavior therapy is the contention that behavior disorder *is* the problem, not just a reflection of the problem. All behavior, normal and abnormal, is learned. The definition of neurosis on which behavior modification rests is that neurotic behavior is the result of learning in the presence of fear- or anxiety-producing stimuli; reversal can be achieved by relearning emotional responses under conditions in which the stimuli are carefully controlled to promote the desired response.[25] Since all behavior is determined by environmental factors, writes Temple University psychologist Alan Goldstein, "behavior therapists absolutely deny the concept of free will in the sense that one ever behaves in a way which is not contingent upon antecedent events."[26]

Consequently, the basic approach in behavior modification or behavior therapy rests on the "laws of learning." Based on laboratory data, it may be simply stated as the likelihood of behavior being repeated if the consequences are perceived as "positive," or suppressed if the consequences are perceived as "negative." Many behaviorists prefer to avoid the popular terms "reward" and "punishment" on the ground that they are value judgments that, like hypothetical constructs, are not observable or measurable. They are also too vague to be good scientific descriptions. (Is the masochist who is subjected to an electric shock being rewarded or punished?)

The central applicable concept of behaviorism is that of *conditioning*. In *classical conditioning*, one of the two major approaches to conditioning, learning is demonstrated by the acquisition of a conditioned response, one that is appropriate to a controlled and predetermined stimulus. Pavlov's dogs responded to classical conditioning. *Operant conditioning* works somewhat differently. It is sometimes referred to as "trial-and-error conditioning," because it is based on a free choice of behaviors. Desirable behavior is "rewarded" or followed by positive reinforcement; undesirable behavior either is "punished" with negative consequences or is ignored.

In operant conditioning, the stimulus actually *follows* the response. For example, a rat may learn to press a bar when he wants food, because pressing the bar is always followed by the dropping of a food pellet into the cage. Because questions of consciousness and motive are avoided, outsiders sometimes have fun trying to decide who is doing what to whom; a cartoon in the *Harvard Crimson*, in the days when Skinner was doing some of his early rat experiments at Harvard, showed a rat leaning against a food lever while saying to another rat, "Boy, do I have this guy trained; every time I press the bar, he drops food into the cage."

Behavior therapy involves a sequence of steps: identification of a response (motor, cognitive, or emotional) that is considered "maladjustive," identification of the circumstances that trigger the unwanted response, and a reconditioning program. The reconditioning program may involve classical conditioning or, more likely, operant conditioning. It may also involve a positive "reinforcement schedule" to make a desired response more likely, or a negative schedule to suppress an unwanted response.

Behaviorists claim that their approach to the treatment of problematic behavior is the only one that is firmly grounded in sound laboratory experimentation and is clearly susceptible to outcome studies. Obviously, if we can define an objective in terms of clearly observable behavior, it would not be difficult to measure and evaluate the degree to which the objective has been achieved.

On the other hand, critics contend that behaviorism is based on a narrow view of human potential and that behavior modification is mechanistic, manipulative, and dehumanizing. S. L. Washburn, professor of anthropology at the University of California at Berkeley and past president of the American Anthropological Association, declared in a related discussion that "human beings are not pigeons who may be taught to peck out the solutions to futile problems. People are the most creative, imaginative, social, empathetic beings that exist."[27] Carl Rogers, a humanist leader, objects that behaviorism does not really describe humans because it fails to recognize the role of "inner" stimuli. "It is quite unfortunate," he writes, "that we have permitted the world of psychological science to be narrowed to behavior observed, sounds emitted, marks scratched on paper, and the like. . . . The inner world of the individual appears to have more significant influence upon his behavior than does the external environmental stimulus."[28]

The heart of the debate focuses on the ability of behaviorism to deal with broad social and personal goals. Arthur W. Combs, a leading spokesman for humanist education, contends that behavioral objectives alone are adequate to deal effectively with such broad humanist goals as self-understanding, self-fulfillment, emotional well-being, and intelligent behavior. During a 1977 debate with behaviorist W. James Popham, Combs made the following statement:

> Such broad, general objectives, having to do with the growth of people as persons, do not lend themselves to description as precisely defined behaviors. If creativity and intelligence could be defined in precise behavioral outcomes, they would not be creative or intelligent. Creativity and intelligent behaviors are outcomes which cannot be foreseen. They are unique human qualities resulting from highly personal, individual interactions between a person and the world in which he or she lives. . . . [O]ur feelings, attitudes, beliefs, loves, hates, hopes, dreams, aspirations, values, and especially our perceptions of ourselves and the world . . . go on inside of people and cannot be dealt with in strictly behavioral terms.[29]

Behaviorists generally concede that there appears to be a public uneasiness about their work, which is often viewed as dehumanizing and manipulative. But, argues Skinner, all people control and are controlled, and all societies establish norms of behavior and punish deviation. The controls exercised by behaviorists are simply more visible — and more effective. Why pretend that an individual has freedom of choice, Skinner asks, when we punish him for violating rules? "Punishable behavior can be minimized," writes Skinner, "by creating circumstances in which it is not likely to occur. . . . [I]t should be possible to design a world in which behavior likely to be punished seldom or never occurs."[30]

The control of human behavior has always been unpopular, Skinner admits, and undisguised efforts to control usually arouse emotional reactions. W. James Popham, who calls himself an "enlightened behaviorist," agrees that "at its least defensible extreme behaviorism represents a dictatorial approach to controlling human actions via a host of effective yet repugnant practices drawn from the animal laboratory. It relies on unbridled operant conditioning to manipulate human beings toward goals they should not have chosen."[31]

And yet, Popham contends, an increasing number of teachers (and it must be recalled that behavior modification is seen as a re-learning process) "will proclaim [their] willingness to judge the quality of an instructional endeavor according to its effects on the behavior of learners."[32]

The major objection to behaviorism is a philosophical one with highly emotional overtones. It is focused on the contention by behaviorists that all behavior is environmentally determined. Skinner called his most controversial book *Beyond Freedom and*

Dignity to make the point that neither word has real meaning; freedom of choice, he argues, is a delusion, since all our actions are nothing but the result of determining influences, genetic or environmental. The prescientific notion of "autonomous" man, which had already been eroded by the work of Marx, Darwin, and Freud, is dismissed as a comforting fiction. Which kind of control is preferable, Skinner asks—that of natural accident or that of social engineering?

Skinner's attack on the concept of autonomous man, as might have been expected, has aroused considerable anger and criticism (which Skinner attributes to wounded vanity). "Although people object when a scientific analysis traces their behavior to external conditions," he contends, "and thus deprives them of credit and the chance to be admired, they seldom object when the same analysis absolves them of blame."[33] Skinner denies that his view is a pessimistic one. Man *can* control his own destiny, since man can modify the determining culture. A scientific view of man, writes Skinner, is an exciting prospect because "we have not yet seen what man can make of man."[34]

Much of the negative press directed at behaviorism has been triggered by reports that have focused on the so-called "aversive" techniques. These techniques are aimed at eliminating specific behaviors by associating with them pain or discomfort, either "real" (physiological, as with electric shock) or "imagined." The aversive techniques do not appear to be in general use in the arts therapies. In fact, a review of the American literature in the expressive therapies discloses that behaviorism itself has not had as significant an impact on these therapies as either psychoanalysis or humanism. Only in music therapy does it seem to play a major role.

For the most part, the arts therapies employ behavior modification techniques only at the lowest levels of operation—with autistic children or the mentally retarded, for example—where the desired responses are rather mechanical, or in areas, such as music, where performance depends largely on the mastery of technical skills.* In these situations, the reinforcement is almost invariably

---

*Perhaps even more important as a reason for the behaviorist orientation in music therapy is the apparent concern of leaders in the field with building a scientifically respectable research base. Of the various psychotherapies, the behavioral is the most amenable to clearly measurable outcome studies. If objectives are defined in terms of observable and measurable behaviors, it is not difficult to ascertain whether or not a therapist or a program has achieved the stated objectives.

"positive," with rewards (smiles, praise, tokens, privileges) offered for desired responses. One specific approach has been adapted from the behaviorist strategies for use in some of the arts therapies — that of "reciprocal inhibition." Patients are taught to inhibit undesired responses by substituting incompatible activities. For example, a movement therapist might train a patient in the technique of deep muscle relaxation or deep diaphragm breathing that he or she can use whenever anxieties or emotions threaten to interfere with effective functioning.

Humanist Therapies: On Becoming More Human

Major differences exist between the broad groups of psychologies (and their associated therapies), known as *existential* and *humanistic*, and there are profound differences *within* each group. It can be confusing to sort out the myriad of new therapies that are often clustered under the humanist umbrella. These therapies range from variant offspring of psychoanalytic theory and applications of existential philosophy to a host of unorthodox therapies like Daniel Casriel's *scream therapy* or Paul Bindrim's *nude marathon*. They include approaches that build on the results of respectable research and those that are frankly and unabashedly antiintellectual and antiscience; proponents of many of the latter group urge their adherents to "feel," to "sense," and to "touch" rather than to think, impelling critics to dub such groups "touchie-feelies."

Despite the differences, however, most of the existential and humanistic approaches rest on shared general assumptions. Virtually all of them are concerned with broadly stated goals, such as helping individuals "to realize their potentials," and they tend to be more focused on growth than on treatment. For purposes of discussion, both the existential and the humanistic approaches will be treated as one broad generalized movement.

These humanistic psychologies have been described as a "third force" between psychoanalysis and behaviorism that rejects the deterministic approaches of both the older schools. (Psychoanalysis stresses the role of inherited instincts and drives, and behaviorism emphasizes the weighty influence of early environment.) The *Articles of Association* of the American Association for Humanistic Psychology defines the thrust of humanist therapy as

> primarily an orientation toward the whole of psychology rather than a distinct area or school. It stands for respect for the worth of persons, respect for differences of approach, open-mindedness as to acceptable methods, an interest in exploration of new aspects of human behavior.

As a "third force" in contemporary psychology it is concerned with topics having little place in existing theories and systems: e.g., love, creativity, self, growth, organism, basic need-gratification, self-actualization, higher values, being, becoming, spontaneity, play, humor, affection, naturalness, warmth, ego-transcendence, objectivity, autonomy, responsibility, meaning, fair-play, transcendental experience, peak experience, courage, and related concepts.[35]

It is difficult to read this statement without being struck by the number of hypothetical constructs with heavy positive emotional connotations. Such constructs as *love, self-actualization,* and *naturalness,* moreover, lend themselves to a wide range of interpretations and to a remarkably wide range of applications, a major reason for the diversity of therapies in the humanistic movement. It is equally apparent from examining this statement that the humanists seek to replace Freudian self-understanding with self-improvement. In fact, the humanistic therapies are therapies only in the broadest sense, since, like behaviorism, they reject the psychoanalytic medical model with its concept of mental illness.

Like the behaviorists, most humanist therapists scoff at the notions that one must search for underlying causes of behavior disorders or trace problems back to their origins. The past is memories, writes Fritz Perls, the father of gestalt therapy, and memories lie. Perls cites Nietzsche, who said, "Memory and Pride were fighting. Memory said, 'It was like this' and Pride said, 'It couldn't have been like this'—and Memory gives in."[36] Perls contends that the great error of psychoanalysis is in assuming that memory is reality:

All the so-called *traumata,* which are supposed to be the root of the neurosis, are an invention of the patient to save his self-esteem. . . . Psychoanalysis fosters the infantile state by considering that the past is responsible for the illness. The patient isn't responsible—no, the trauma is responsible, or the Oedipus complex is responsible, and so on. . . . We have got such an idea about the importance of this invented memory, where the whole illness is supposed to be based on this memory. No wonder that all the wild goose chase of the psychoanalyst to find out *why* I am now like this can never come to an end, can never prove a real opening up by the person himself. . . . *Why* and *because* are dirty words in Gestalt Therapy. They lead only to rationalization.[37]

The key words in humanism are *here* and *now.* Few problems that exist in the present, declares Abraham Maslow, are so similar to those of the past that we can apply past solutions.[38] In dealing with the problems of the *here* and *now,* the focus is on *feeling* rather than *thinking.* At the heart of humanism are the concepts of self-improvement and personal growth; the stress is on educating and helping individuals to attain their unique potentialities and on working toward *self-actualization,* or *individuation,* or *self-development.* Whereas psychoanalysis and behaviorism adhere to the concept of normality, the humanist thinks of "positive" behavior in terms of the unique attributes and potential of an individual. To Maslow, normality is "a psychopathology of the average . . . [a] general phoniness . . . living by illusions and by fear."[39] Since humanism is more readily perceived in educational rather than in therapeutic (medical) terms, the role of the therapist-healer is minimized (in many groups, the therapist is a "facilitator") or even abolished. Such approaches lend themselves to popularization and inevitably to the development of a host of self-help offshoots.

It is difficult to describe humanism with any kind of precision, partly because of the great variety of therapies that are encompassed by the term and partly because of the reluctance of most humanists to circumscribe their possibilities by over-precise definitions or standards or descriptions. There is a great fear that the kind of orthodoxy might develop that humanists see in classical Freudian psychoanalysis. However, an examination of gestalt therapy, probably the best known of the humanistic or self-growth therapies, reveals much that is common to humanism.

Gestalt therapy bears only a tenuous relationship to the psychology of the same name that developed in Germany in the early days of the twentieth century. *Gestalt,* in German, means *form* or *configuration* (not "whole," as is generally assumed), and the psychology was based on an interest in the ways in which humans perceive the world in which they live. In particular, the gestalt psychologists were intrigued with the human tendency to see patterns, to complete pictures from fragmentary data, to "make whole." For obvious reasons, gestalt psychology was of considerable interest to artists, and some elements of the original psychology can be found in the work of gestalt art therapists.

Gestalt *therapy* is largely the creation of Frederick S. (Fritz) Perls, a German-born psychoanalyst with both M.D. and Ph.D. degrees, who came to view traditional psychoanalysis with contempt. He rejected the idea of the unconscious and dismissed the theory of repression. Increasingly, Perls's work at the Esalen Institute in California came to focus on the concrete and the obvious, rather than the abstract, and he stressed the need to deal with immediate problems and present solutions. Perls saw disturbed or disturbing behavior as a symptom of polarization between conflicting psychological elements; the therapeutic treatment consists of bringing the discordant elements into a mutual self-disclosing confrontation.

The fundamental relationship between gestalt therapy and the psychology from which it derived its name is on the shared concept of "completion." Gestalt therapy seeks, in Perls's words, "to fill in the holes in the personality to make the person whole and complete again."[40] Gestalt therapy can be used with individuals, but is more frequently conducted in group sessions, with the therapist taking an active—and highly directive—role. (In this respect, gestalt therapy differs from the approach in many of the humanist therapies in which the therapist is a nondirective "facilitator.")

Perls's own personality has shaped the role model for gestalt therapists, a development that is deplored by some of the leaders in the field. Walter Kempler, a former collaborator who broke with Perls on the issue of the conduct of therapy sessions, insists that a distinction should be made between Perls's personal "hot-seat" approach (which Kempler attributes to Perls's psychoanalytic training), in which Perls always maintained a top-dog attitude toward his patients, and the psychological model called gestalt therapy.[41] However, Perls's own writings remain, to date, the prevailing statements of gestalt therapy, despite the fact that they provide limited theoretical structure. As a result, what occasionally seems to prevail on the pseudogestalt scene, as distinguished from the responsible practice of gestalt therapy, is the development of what has come to be known as "psycho-babble" (being "at," coming "from," getting your head together) as a substitute for a coherent philosophy or a psychological structure. Part of the problem springs from the fact that the Gestalt Training Institutes that mushroomed after Perls's death in 1970 are locally autonomous and adhere to varied standards of training and certification for therapists. Since a strong spirit prevails in the movement to defy standardization, it is not likely that uniformity of standards is forthcoming in the near future.

Kempler and other pioneers in humanism worry about the susceptibility of humanism in general to encroachment by the "gimmick therapist," who has seized upon the growing popularity of the movement. The gimmick therapist, whom he also calls the "tactician," is the greatest hazard to the movement, contends Kempler, because of "the loss of vitality that comes from trying to become a disciple of a method rather than using the principles of the method."[42] Kempler sees the roots of the problem, at least in gestalt therapy, as the subjective nature of gestalt philosophy, the absence of sound, well-organized theory, and the difficulty of encouraging people to be themselves while at the same time maintaining standards of competence for therapists.

The problem of marginally competent practitioners in gestalt therapy has grown since Perls's death. However, he himself had been uncomfortably aware of the developing problem even during his life. In the introduction to *Gestalt Therapy Verbatim*, he complained that gestalt therapy was entering the phase of "the turner-onners . . . the quacks and the con-men," who use technique and gimmicks. The sad fact, he warned, "is that this jazzing-up more often becomes a dangerous substitute activity, another phony therapy that *prevents* growth."[43]

The popularization of humanistic theories and practices has led in some quarters to the debasement and adulteration of the ideas of the founders. For example, Perls's well-known motto "Lose your mind and come to your senses" was a dramatic way of suggesting that thinking itself might interfere with the attempt to identify one's feelings. Perls himself, however, was not antiintellectual; he saw clearly the value of thinking that is directed toward a purpose, such as problem solving. Most people, he contended, use "thinking" for rationalization, to fantasize scenarios in which they "rehearse" the roles they intend to play with others in order to impress them. For most individuals, therefore, thinking is a form of avoidance, a way of insulating oneself against the impact of real feelings. In many of the "touchie-feelie" therapies that have sprouted around the edges of humanism, the exhortation to expose oneself to feeling has been converted into a mindless and narcissistic flight from reason.

The problem of maintaining standards in a movement whose very philosophy resists limitation is admittedly difficult, and the infiltration of the movement by the gimmick therapists may be impossible to control. In the introduction to *Existential Psychology*, Rollo May pleaded that the whole movement not be smeared by the behavior of some of its practitioners; he quoted Nietzsche's aphorism: "The . . . adherents of a movement are no argument against it."[44]

Gestalt therapy, of course, is only one of the therapies that are generally referred to as humanistic. And Perls himself owed much of his theory to others, many of whom founded psychologies and therapies that are loosely associated with the humanistic movement. In particular, Perls's view of the human organism as a whole, rather than a combination of parts, owes much to the work of Wilhelm Reich. Reich had a profound influence on the humanistic movement in general, and his ideas stimulated the development of a group of therapies referred to as *body therapies*. Reich had studied with Freud and for a time had been a traditional Freudian analyst. Like so many of Freud's followers, he broke with Freud to found his own psychology and to develop a related therapy.

Reich observed that physical tensions frequently accompany other signs of mental distress, and he formulated the theory that *character resistance* is expressed in the body as well as the mind. *Body armor* and *muscular armor* are terms that Reich used to describe the creation of muscular tension blocks and armor as defenses against threatening situations. Faced with hostile or threatening possibilities, for example, people hold their breaths and tighten their muscles; however, while such rigidity may protect the physical person (often it is self-defeating), it inhibits the free flow of emotional energy. Muscular tension and emotional repression, Reich hypothesized, are symptoms of the same problem. By freeing the muscular tensions, he argued, he could dissolve the neurosis.[45]

Unfortunately for his hypotheses, Reich also formulated a number of rather bizarre theories that discredited him among serious psychologists. For example, he expanded Freud's concept of psychic energy into the idea of *orgones* — floating particles of energy that could be trapped in a box in which a patient sat. Reich died in prison, where he had been sent for fraud involving the sale of orgone boxes. Related work by researchers and practitioners, however, has revived the Reichian concept of *characterological armor*. It was found that physical activity often promotes deeper emotional release than does verbal expression and that there are, indeed, relationships between physical manifestation and emotional state. As a result, a host of body therapies have developed, some of which appear to have a firm foundation in research — and many of which do not.

One of the major spokesmen for the body therapies is Alexander Lowen, the founder of *bioenergetics*, who contends that a trained bioenergetic therapist can make a "character analysis" of an individual by an examination of that person's body. Lowen claims that the blocked emotional feelings of an individual are manifested in his or her muscular pattern. Moreover, he asserts, not only do the emotions shape anatomy, distorting posture and knotting muscles, but physical behavior influences an individual's mental state.[46] As a result, therapy in bioenergetics is perhaps more physical than it is verbal.

The physical and nonverbal aspects of the body therapies have been seized upon eagerly by many (but by no means all) of the humanistic therapies, which frequently combine verbal and non-verbal approaches, on the ground that the nonverbal act is in itself a combination of communication, exploration, self-awareness, and therapy.

The influence of the humanistic psychologies on the expressive arts therapies has been profound. For one thing, the arts involve symbolic expression and nonverbal communication; they focus on self-expression and identity. The therapeutic act and the creative act are merged into the process that is variously described as *self-actualization*[47] and *individuation*,[48] as the individual comes increasingly in touch with inner feelings and perceptions in the process of expressing them. For this reason, the concept of *authenticity* is as central to the practice of humanistic therapies as it is in psychoanalysis.

Because both behaviorists and humanists reject the medical model, both groups tend to view their own practice in terms of education at least as much as therapy. However, the refusal of humanists to deal with narrow "operational" goals has drawn the scorn of behaviorists like Popham:

> When we think about humanism the vibrations are invariably positive. The majority of humanists endorse the kinds of values that most of us praise. And it is difficult to think ill of those who defend such praiseworthy, if ill-defined, intentions as "helping [individuals] achieve their full human and social potentials."[49]

But, Popham contends, there are many abysmally weak educational — and presumably therapeutic — programs "now comfortably nestled behind such humanist slogans." Humanists have it easy, he argues, when they refuse to "put their effectiveness on the line. Since they function in ethereal realms," because they claim that behavioral evidence is inadequate for their purposes, "no one can tie them down. Instructional travesties will prosper alongside instructional triumphs."[50]

The humanist movement is still in its formative stages. At this time, it is still too early to ascertain the ways or the extent to which criticism from the outside — and self-criticism by leaders within the movement — will affect the future development of humanism.

WHAT WORKS IN PSYCHOTHERAPY?

While the three groupings discussed in this chapter are umbrellas for the bulk of the therapies practiced in this country, there are dozens of therapies that cannot be classified within these categories. (Some of them, of course, are therapies in name only, being little more than activities that are deemed "therapeutic," such as ballroom dancing, gardening, or casting plaster wall plaques, or exercises and routines that are conducted uniformly for all participants, without regard for individual diagnoses or needs.) Most therapists, it would appear, practice some form of "eclectic" therapy, drawing ideas and techniques from related therapies if they appear to enhance the possibilities of achieving the desired goals. The gimmick therapist, of whom Perls, Kempler, and others complain, borrows indiscriminately, without regard to the problems of the patient, without goals, and without a consistent theoretical structure or plan of treatment; the gimmick therapist is using a bag of tricks.

Can one make sense of the babel of claims and counterclaims? Which of the therapies is the gold, and which the dross? Indeed, do *any* of the therapies really work?

The evidence is not clear, but patterns are beginning to emerge. Earlier studies, and some recent ones as well, suggest not only that there is no significant difference in the efficacy of one form of therapy over another, but that the improvement rate of neurotic patients undergoing psychotherapy tends to be no higher than that of untreated individuals on waiting lists. More recent research shows, however, that the latter conclusion is an oversimplification. During the 1970s, Lester Luborsky of the University of Pennsylvania conducted a massive review of the literature in psychotherapy and amassed data on a large number of outcome studies. This overview failed to support the superiority of one form of psychotherapy over another. One major conclusion did stand out, though: psychotherapy does work — sometimes and with some patients.[51]

What makes it work? The research findings to date are insufficient to provide a simple, clear answer, but some tentative discoveries are suggestive. Four factors, in particular, seem to be influential in determining whether psychotherapy will work.

The severity of the disorder. The more severe the problem, the smaller the likelihood of success in treatment. Considerable evidence indicates that *neuroses* (or *anxiety disorders*, as they are now called in the latest manual of the American Psychiatric Association) tend to be self-limiting; time alone will alleviate or cure most of them, as it does most colds or bruises.[52] At the other end of the scale, severely disordered psychotics seem to be the least helped by any form of psychotherapy. In fact, only in the United States is psychotherapy still occasionally employed as a primary treatment for schizophrenia; almost everywhere else in the world, it has been abandoned in favor of chemotherapy, the use of anti-psychotic drugs.[53]

The educational and social level of the patient. The over-whelming bulk of psychotherapy is verbal. As has often been noted, psychotherapy is a talking cure — sometimes referred to as "healing by conversation." Not only do the more educated patients share a belief in the value of psychotherapy (more on this follows), but they tend to be more verbal than poorly educated patients. They can communicate with the therapist, and they share with the therapist, more-over, a faith in the value of words to describe, express, and control experiences.

The patient's faith in the efficacy of the treatment. Patients may seek out therapists of a particular theoretical persuasion, or they may go from therapist to therapist until they find one who "helps" them. For the most part, the decision to stay with a therapist seems to have more to do with an emotional affinity — with the approach as well as with the therapist — than with the logic of the underlying theory. A patient, for example, may find terrifying the existential thought that all of life's meaning exists in this moment; conversely, another may find equally frightening the Freudian view that his or her childhood experiences cast a shadow over present and future. Some researchers hypothesize that the secret of success in psy-chotherapy is suggestion and that the patient who shares the "myth" of the efficacy of a particular brand of therapy (or the competence of a therapist) is likely to show the greatest improve-ment.[54] Dr. E. Fuller Torrey, a psychiatrist who has studied healing in primitive societies, claims that medicine men obtain about the same degree of success among their patients as psychotherapists do among theirs.[55] Apparently, the therapist's faith in his or her own method is a major factor in successful therapy; this faith is communicated to the patient.

The relationship between therapist and patient. Substantial evi-dence demonstrates that when therapist and patient like and respect each other — usually for reasons that have little to do with the spe-cific psychotherapeutic method used — the therapy is likely to be more successful than when they do not like each other. A number of researchers argue that personality is a more important influence on the success of psychotherapy than the therapist's academic creden-tials or the specific method of treatment. "To care for people," writes Harry Guntrip, "is more important than to care for ideas."[56]

A closely related element in successful therapy is the willingness of the therapist to shape the program to the needs of the patient rather than the structure of the method. Reviewing the various approaches to psychoanalysis, R. L. Munroe states flatly: "All good analytic work is actually centered around the patient, not around a theory."[57]

The theoretical parameters, however, do help to shape the relationship between therapist and patient and to enhance or diminish the importance of the therapist's personality. Reviewing evidence from research studies and from clinical observation, Allen E. Bergin and Hans H. Strupp conclude that the personality of the therapist is most important in client-centered therapy and least important in behavior therapy, although they admit that it is not clear how therapist personality and technical operations can be differentiated.[58]

IMPLICATIONS FOR RESEARCH IN THE ARTS THERAPIES

The arts therapies are infant professions-in-the-making, and the research on what works in these therapies is even sketchier than is psychotherapy. There is some reason to believe that many patients who are unresponsive to the talking cure may be reached by nonverbal approaches. Dance therapy pioneer Marian Chace concluded from her own experiences that nonverbal approaches may be the only way of communicating with severely regressed patients who are "locked in a world of silence."[59] Such nonverbal approaches may also open doors to communication with poorly educated or generally nonverbal patients.

For the most part, though, such views about the value of the arts therapies remain untested hypotheses. The expressive therapies have been largely ignored by researchers in psychotherapy. For example, *The Therapist's Handbook*, a "multidisciplinary" compilation by twenty-eight authorities in the field of mental health, provides some testimony on the disregard by verbal therapists for the nonverbal therapies. The index has not a single entry under art, dance, music, movement, body, or soma. (Psychosomatic disorders, on the other hand, are dealt with in seventy-four pages of the work, a clear indication of how the contributors view the relationship between mind and body.) The one reference to *somatic therapies* (pp. 307–08) deals with electric convulsive therapy, vitamins, and psychosurgery.[60] It is not likely that meaningful research on the value of the nonverbal therapies will come from the ranks of psychotherapists.

Practitioners in the arts therapies themselves have been slow in developing programs of self-evaluation or of investigation of the outcome of treatment. They have been too busy struggling for acceptance in the mental health establishment, developing theoretical bases (often from psychotherapy), and establishing standards for training and practice.

The value of theory should not be underestimated. It has been pointed out that in psychotherapy, theoretical considerations are less important in the success of a program than the characteristics of patient and therapist. Nevertheless, a coherent theoretical structure provides a plan of action. Without it, the therapist has no guidelines, no way of knowing how an activity, a tactic, or a technique fits into a general approach, or even if it has any value in the specific program; each experience exists in isolation, with no connection to those that preceded it or to those that will follow.

The value of any therapy, however, rests less on the logic of its theoretical structure than on the answer to the question, how well does it succeed in doing what it purports to do? Unless theoretical formulations are actually tested in practice under controlled conditions, there is no way of knowing what actually works. Except for some limited work in music therapy (where, unfortunately, the behavioral objectives are still too narrowly conceived to answer the question about how well the programs achieve their major overriding goals), there is a remarkable paucity of solid data on what works in nonverbal therapy. The general inclination has been to rest on the research work that has been done in the psychotherapies — a shaky platform on which to build. Until research in the therapies catches up with practice and theory building, it will be difficult to assess the effectiveness of any psychotherapeutic theory in its application to the arts therapies. Currently, all of them find adherents in these fields. An increasing number of expressive arts therapists have begun to wonder aloud if, in the absence of solid outcome research in the psychotherapies, the expressive therapies should not develop independent theoretical structures.

REFERENCE NOTES

1. Hans J. Eysenck, "The Effects of Psychotherapy," *International Journal of Psychotherapy* 1 (1965), quoted in Martin L. Gross, *The Psychological Society* (New York: Random House, 1978), p. 23.
2. Ibid.
3. Gross, *The Psychological Society*, p. 55.

4. Arnold A. Rogow, *The Psychiatrists* (New York: G. P. Putnam's Sons, 1970).
5. Sigmund Freud, *The Question of Lay Analysis: Conversations with an Impartial Person*, trans. James Strachey (New York: W. W. Norton, 1969).
6. Sigmund Freud, *New Introductory Lectures in Psychoanalysis*, trans. W. J. H. Sprott (New York: W. W. Norton, 1935), pp. 103-05.
7. Sigmund Freud, *The Psychopathology of Everyday Life*, trans. A. A. Brill (London: Ernest Benn, 1935), p. 63.
8. June Singer, *Boundaries of the Soul: The Practice of Jung's Psychology* (Garden City, N.Y.: Doubleday, Anchor Books, 1972), p. 85.
9. Carl G. Jung, *Man and His Symbols* (Garden City, N.Y.: Doubleday, 1964), pp. 20-21.
10. E. C. Whitmont and Yoram Kaufmann, "Analytical Psychotherapy," in *Current Psychotherapies*, ed. Raymond Corsini (Itasca, Ill.: F. E. Peacock, 1973), p. 90.
11. Jung, *Man and His Symbols*, p. 24.
12. Carl G. Jung, *The Integration of the Personality* (New York: Farrar and Rinehart, 1939), quoted in Donn Byrne, *An Introduction to Personality*, 2nd ed. (Englewood Cliffs, N.J.: Prentice-Hall, 1974), p. 46.
13. Carl G. Jung, *Memories, Dreams, Reflections* (New York: Vintage Books, 1965), p. 196.
14. Alfred Adler, *What Life Should Mean to You* (New York: Capricorn Books, 1958), p. 72.
15. Albert Ellis, "Humanism, Values, Rationality," *Journal of Individual Psychology* 26 (1970):37-38.
16. Byrne, *An Introduction to Personality*, p. 52.
17. Robert P. Knight, *Clinician and Therapist: Selected Papers of Robert P. Knight*, ed. Stuart C. Miller (New York: Basic Books, 1972), p. 13.
18. E. Fuller Torrey, *The Death of Psychiatry* (New York: Penguin Books, 1975).
19. Christopher Lasch, "Sacrificing Freud," *New York Times Magazine*, February 22, 1976, p. 11.
20. Ibid.
21. Letter to *APA Monitor*, quoted in Daniel Goleman, "Who's Mentally Ill?" *Psychology Today* 11, no. 8 (January 1978):34.
22. John B. Watson, "Psychology as the Behaviorist Views It," *Psychological Review* 20 (1913):158-77.
23. Gerald Jonas, *Visceral Learning: Toward a Science of Self-Control* (New York: The Viking Press, 1973), p. 137.
24. Arthur Bandura, *Principles of Behavior Modification* (New York: Holt, Rinehart and Winston, 1969); Alan E. Kazdin, *Behavior Modification in Applied Settings* (Homewood, Ill.: The Dorsey Press, 1975).
25. J. Wolpe, *Psychotherapy by Reciprocal Inhibition* (Stanford, Calif.: Stanford University Press, 1959).
26. Alan Goldstein, "Behavior Therapy," in Corsini, *Current Psychotherapies*, p. 219.

27. S. L. Washburn, "Evaluation and Learning," *National Elementary Principal* 54, no. 6 (July/August 1975):6.
28. Carl R. Rogers, "Toward a Science of the Person," in *Behaviorism and Phenomenology: Contrasting Bases for Modern Psychology*, ed. T. W. Wann (Chicago: University of Chicago Press, 1964), pp. 118, 125.
29. Arthur W. Combs, "A Humanist's View," *Educational Leadership* 35, no. 1 (October 1977):55.
30. B. F. Skinner, *Beyond Freedom and Dignity* (New York: Bantam Books/ Vintage, 1971), p. 60.
31. W. James Popham, "Behaviorism as a Bugbear," *Educational Leadership* 35, no. 1 (October 1977):57.
32. Ibid.
33. Skinner, *Beyond Freedom and Dignity*, p. 71.
34. Ibid., p. 206.
35. F. T. Severin, *Humanistic Viewpoints in Psychology* (New York: McGraw-Hill, 1965), pp. xv-xvi.
36. Frederick S. Perls, *Gestalt Therapy Verbatim* (Lafayette, Calif.: Real People Press, 1969; New York: Bantam Books, 1971), p. 45.
37. Ibid., pp. 46-47.
38. Abraham Maslow, "The Creative Attitude," *The Structurist* 3 (1963):4-10, reprinted in *The Helping Relationship*, eds. Donald L. Avila, Arthur W. Combs, and William W. Purkey (Boston: Allyn and Bacon, 1975), p. 389.
39. Abraham Maslow, "Existential Psychology—What's In It for Us?" in *Existential Psychology*, ed. Rollo May (New York: Random House, 1961), p. 60.
40. Perls, *Gestalt Therapy Verbatim*, p. 2.
41. Walter Kempler, "Gestalt Therapy," in *Current Psychotherapies*, p. 254.
42. Ibid.
43. Perls, *Gestalt Therapy Verbatim*, p. 1.
44. May, *Existential Psychology*.
45. Wilhelm Reich, *Character Analysis* (New York: Orgone Institute Press, 1944).
46. Alexander Lowen, *The Language of the Body* (New York: Collier Books, 1958).
47. Abraham Maslow, *Toward a Psychology of Being* (New York: Van Nostrand Reinhold Co., 1968).
48. Carl Rogers, *On Becoming a Person* (Boston: Houghton Mifflin Co., 1961).
49. Popham, "Behaviorism as a Bugbear," p. 61.
50. Ibid.
51. Lester Luborsky, "Comparative Studies of Psychotherapies," *Archives of General Psychiatry* 32 (1975):995-1008.
52. Louis A. Gottschalk et al., "A Study of Prediction and Outcome in a Mental Health Crisis Clinic," *American Journal of Psychiatry* 130, no. 10 (October 1973):1107-11.
53. E. Fuller Torrey, "Tracing the Causes of Madness," *Psychology Today* 12, no. 10 (March 1979):79.

54. Kenneth M. Calestro, "Psychotherapy, Faith Healing and Suggestion," *International Journal of Psychiatry* 10 (1972):83–113.
55. E. Fuller Torrey, *The Mind Game: Witchdoctors and Psychiatrists* (New York: Emerson Books, 1972).
56. Harry Guntrip, *Psychoanalytic Theory, Therapy and the Self* (New York: Basic Books, 1973), p. v., quoted in Samuel B. Kutash, "Modified Psychoanalytic Therapies," in *The Therapist's Handbook*, ed. B. Wolman (New York: Van Nostrand Reinhold, 1976), p. 89.
57. R. L. Munroe, *Schools of Psychoanalytic Thought* (New York: Dryden Press, 1955), p. 507.
58. Allen E. Bergin and Hans H. Strupp, *Changing Frontiers in the Science of Psychotherapy* (Chicago and New York: Aldine-Atherton, 1972), pp. 24–29.
59. *Marian Chace: Her Papers*, ed., Harris Chaiklin (Columbia, Md.: American Dance Therapy Association, 1975), p. 44.
60. Benjamin B. Wolman, ed., *The Therapist's Handbook: Treatment Methods of Mental Disorders* (New York: Van Nostrand Reinhold, 1976).

3

Visual Arts Therapy

Metaphoric clichés may be considered the free associations of a culture. The remarkable frequency of color terms in clichés that are used to describe personality suggests that our perception of personality is emotionally colored, in the most literal sense. Adjectives used to describe emotion are often color coded. You may be green with envy, red with rage, purple with passion; everything may look black when you suffer the blues, or, in contrast, you may see the world through rose-colored glasses. Color is an obvious and simple way to organize our feelings—and ultimately our thinking—about the world in general. Indeed, researchers point out that color discrimination is one of the earliest ways in which children classify objects.[1]

Color and the more sophisticated elements of form and shape are the components of the images that we perceive and that we create as we build our mental models of the world. According to developmental psychologists Jean Piaget and Jerome Bruner, image making is a major stage in cognitive development.[2] Color is the element that appears to be more closely associated with emotion, while form and shape seem to be related to thought.

To the ancient Greeks, such a distinction might have made little sense; just as they recognized the unity of body and mind, the Greeks perceived the interrelationship between emotion — the language of the soul — and thought. Aristotle, that prolific commentator on the universe, once noted that "the soul never thinks without an image," a statement that must have made sense in the most literal terms to the ancients, to whom dreams and visions were messages — from the gods, from the spirits, from the cosmos.

Modern Westerners have tended to view such statements as metaphor — if, indeed, they even accepted the notion of soul. Freud once again made respectable the view that dreams and images are messages, but messages of emotion, rather than thought, and messages *from* the soul itself, which Freud termed the unconscious. Dreams, to Freud, were the surfacing of feelings, instinctual urges, and repressed emotions from that "seething cauldron of excitement."

In the Western scientific tradition, however, most speculation about humans rests on a peculiar binary assumption: that all human activity is *either-or*. So even as Freud's postulate gained wide acceptance, images were relegated to a subordinate message center. *Thinking*, in contrast with *feeling*, was a function of language; a large verbal vocabulary has been the distinguishing feature of the intelligent (and educated) man or woman.

Just as the old body-mind dichotomy has been brought under scrutiny in recent years, so too have the reason-emotion and word-image distinctions. In his book *Visual Thinking*, Rudolf Arnheim, Professor Emeritus of the psychology of art at Harvard, argues convincingly that all thinking is perceptual in nature. He contends that perception involves an ordering of experience and a structuring of events. In the act of perception itself, we organize and classify events and objects. Even abstract reasoning, he asserts, involves imagery on the diagrammatic and the symbolic levels.[3] Emotion itself, he claims, is a *function* of perception.[4]

However, despite increasing evidence that the old dichotomies are based on simpleminded views of the world, these either-or distinctions still dominate much of our commonsense thinking.

Not only have emotion and reason been divorced, but they have been provided with separate homes; we may obey the dictates of our heads *or* our hearts. Such divisions still underlie much of the theory and practice of the psychotherapies. It is conceded that emotional problems will affect and influence an individual's thinking, but the resolution almost always is cognitive. In psychoanalysis, the resolution of emotional problems usually involves the re-*cognition* of a problem — which must almost always be verbalized.

The expressive arts therapies often blur these psychotherapeutic distinctions. While the arts therapies have adopted the terms and classification systems of the psychotherapies, implicit in much of the practice is the assumption that a human being is a unitary and indivisible organism. This is one reason (by no means the only one, as we shall see later) that so much of the arts therapies' technique, if not necessarily their theories, are compatible with much of humanism. One major convergence between the arts therapies and at least some of the humanistic approaches is the general, but not universal, assumption that thinking and creativity are related.* The weighing of the influence of creativity in art therapy is the source of much of the confusion over definitions in the new field.

The official definition of art therapy adopted by the American Art Therapy Association (AATA) reads as follows:

> Within the field of art therapy there are two major approaches.
>
> The use of art as therapy implies that the creative process can be a means both of reconciling conflicts and of fostering self-awareness and personal growth.
>
> When using art as a vehicle for psychotherapy, both the product and the associative references may be used in an effort to help the individual find a more compatible relationship between his inner and outer worlds.[5]

This definition would appear to bow in the direction of humanists and psychoanalytically oriented practitioners. However, at the

---

*Except for a few "nonverbal" tests for illiterates and for very young children, the bulk of our intelligence tests are composed of words. The vast majority of them perpetuate the distinction between creativity and intelligence by excluding from the factors of intelligence such characteristics as originality and persistence, or any form of divergent thinking. Normally, these characteristics are seen as attributes of "personality," which is clearly distinguished from "intelligence." For a more complete discussion of the issues involved in the debate over IQ tests, see Chapter 2 of Bernard Feder, *The Complete Guide to Taking Tests* (Englewood Cliffs, N.J.: Prentice-Hall, 1979).

local levels, and within the ranks of the national association itself, proffered alternative definitions are banners displaying the variety and strength of various theoretical affiliations. For example, the Maryland Art Therapy Association, in an undated and unpaginated pamphlet, presents art therapy as "a new dimension in self-expression and expanded self-awareness, and catharsis," which provides opportunities to explore "alternative options through creative artistic channels," and which "links the imagination factor to conscious decision making."

The remarkable diversity of backgrounds and psychological biases among art therapists helps to explain the wide range of definitions offered by practitioners, an embarrassment of riches that is the despair of some, the delight of others. Edith Wallace, a Jungian analyst, told an audience at the 1976 convention of the AATA that "the beauty of art therapy is that in the last analysis it is not definable, in the same way that the creative process — no matter how much we can and do say about it — is ultimately a mystery." But, she added wryly, "Try telling that to the accrediting authorities."[6]

Nevertheless, implicit in most of the definitions is the agreement that the emerging field deals with creative impulses and emotional expression. The relative mix of these elements is the subject of an intense debate in the field. The two directions from which art therapists approach the discipline — *art* and *therapy* — and the emphasis that practitioners choose to put on one of them help to determine the functions of art therapy for the individual practitioner.

To varying degrees, each of the art functions — diagnostic and therapeutic — discussed in this chapter stresses one of the two poles: *creative production* and *expressive communication*. However, just as there is an overlap in creativity and communication, there is also an overlap in functions.

THE DIAGNOSTIC USE OF ART

When Sigmund Freud unlocked the door to the unconscious and wrote of the images presented in dreams, he gave art therapists a solid base for diagnostic work that follows and parallels psychoanalytic processes. Freud himself pointed out that "all of our dreams are preponderantly visual,"[7] and he was painfully aware that much of the dream experience is lost in the translation of these images into words. If an art product is seen as a "frozen fragment of a dream" — a common expression among art therapists, suggesting that a dream-image has been preserved for diagnosis — then the art therapist's work involves a process that may be more direct than that of the psychoanalyst. Whereas the verbal therapist must deal with translations of dream-images, the art therapist can deal with reproductions of the images. Freud noted that his patients frequently said that they could draw an image, but that they were unable to describe it in words.[8]

Margaret Naumburg, a Freudian-oriented pioneer in art therapy, writes that "although Freud made the modern world aware that the unconscious speaks in images, he did not follow the suggestion of his patients that they be permitted to draw their dreams, rather than to tell them."[9] In fact, Freud insisted that the images be verbalized,[10] apparently on the ground that verbal expression is indispensable to the communication of a problem and to its resolution. Some psychoanalysts, however, believe that there are significant differences between thinking and communicating in images and doing so in words.

Psychiatrist Mardi J. Horowitz of San Francisco's Mount Zion Medical Center thinks that visual image making may be superior to verbal communication in many situations. "Some types of information," he says, "may be expressed and communicated in images better than in words." Many childhood memories, and even repressed memories and fantasies, "are accessible to consciousness in image representation, but are inexpressible in words, since they cannot be translated into verbal form."[11] Moreover, the expression through pictures is much more symbolic and less specific than is expression through words. Memories and fantasies may emerge in the process of drawing without the patient's awareness of what is being disclosed and with less likelihood of censorship. The communication may be less explicit than it would be in verbal therapy — for example, the patient need not acknowledge that the family in a drawing is his or her family. Because such protecting devices are built into the art therapy process, the expression — and communication — of feelings is less threatening and therefore less likely than verbal therapy to invite suppression and intellectualization.

Not only specific content, but general patterns of content may have diagnostic value. Jolande Jacobi, for example, has found common recurrent features in the work of obsessional neurotics that include stereotypes — motifs from the genital and urinary areas, and motifs that show a sort of grill or crossbar pattern — which suggest to Jacobi a psychic blockage pattern.[12]

In addition to the content of an image, the form in which the image is created may reveal much about the patient. Naumburg writes:

> Some spontaneous pictures created by patients show imaged patterns of response that are typical of specific mental illnesses. Schizophrenic thinking is, for instance, frequently expressed in the fragmented forms of certain pictures. A schizophrenic design, when explained by a patient, often uses a single image to represent an elaborate sequence of ideas. . . . Clearly diagnostic elements are frequently evident in the rigid geometric patterns of paranoid images. There is usually much black in the pictures of severely regressed patients. . . . Another diagnostic element frequently found in the spontaneous images created by patients during art therapy is symbolic expression of either regression or progression in the therapeutic process. Changes in a series of symbolic images frequently inform the art therapist of positive changes in the course of a patient's treatment.[13]

An impressive number of diagnostic clues center on the representation of the body. Psychotic patients often have a distorted image of their own bodies, a phenomenon that is the basis for much of the work done in dance/movement therapy (see Chapter 5). This confusion in body image is often displayed as well in the drawings that such patients create. Such distortions are quite distinguishable from those that result from intellectual retardation or just poor drawing ability. Commenting on a primitive human figure drawn by a twelve-year-old retarded boy, Emery I. Gondor of New York Medical College notes that "the mouth represented, like the eye, by a circle, is drawn outside and below the face. . . . The emptiness and the confusion of the body image in the drawing indicate that in addition to the retardation, we are dealing with a psychotic disturbance, which was later confirmed by medical examination."[14]

Individual body features may provide clues to specific disturbances. Dr. Paul Jay Fink, then of Hahnemann Medical College and Hospital in Philadelphia, asserts that menacing eyes "usually indicate paranoia," but he warns that the therapist "must learn to discriminate paranoid eyes from those which are softer, less menacing, and less probing."[15]

While humanist art therapists tend to discount the medical model, with its classifications of psychopathology, they too see value in art products as indicators of a client's underlying view of the world — and of the individual's place in it. "The way we perceive visually," writes Janie Rhyne, "is directly related to how we think and feel."[16] The emergence of central figures from the background, the use of line, color, shape, structure, and space, humanist therapists believe, are indicative of the ways an individual patterns his or her life.

Up to this point, we have been discussing the use of spontaneously produced images for diagnostic purposes. In a very different category is the diagnostic use of already created pictures, as in the Rosenzweig Picture-Frustration Study, or in the Thematic Apperception Test (TAT) (see *A Tool of the Trade*, p. 89), or in the use of prepared nonrepresentational materials as in the Rorschach Test (see *A Tool of the Trade*, p. 90). Such materials are often based on the Freudian concept of *projection*: the tendency of individuals to externalize, that is, to ascribe to others the drives, feelings, and instincts that they themselves experience.

Projective techniques are often used in the interpretation of spontaneously produced materials, but they are the primary thrust of many of the so-called test approaches. The projective tests are based not only on the notion of projection, but on the attempt to provide patients with standard tasks, so that comparisons can be made between "normal" and "abnormal" responses. Obviously, it would be difficult to standardize the task involved in creating a spontaneous drawing, so most of the projective tests provide uniform prompting devices to elicit verbal responses. In fact, they are often used by clinical psychologists who have had no training at all in art. As a result, many art therapists consider them techniques in verbal therapy (actually diagnosis) rather than legitimate applications of art therapy techniques.

Bernard I. Levy, chairing a symposium of leading art therapists at the general session of the fifth annual AATA convention, may well have had such techniques in mind when he asserted: "Art therapy is a unique enterprise, distinct from both verbal psychotherapy and activity group therapy. Art therapy must not be regarded as a back door into the practice of other forms of psychotherapy."[17]

On the other hand, proponents of such projective test approaches point out that the spontaneously drawn image that is the basis for most art therapy diagnosis is not as direct a representation of a dream or a fantasy as is often assumed; drawing requires a translation of mind pictures into a form in which much significant detail or nuance may be lost. A major drawback of the projective response approaches, in the eyes of many art therapists, is that they cannot be used to elicit authentic responses that are uncued and open.

According to reviewers of projective techniques in the *Mental Measurements Yearbooks*,[18] most are interpreted psychoanalytically.

Visual stimuli are often viewed as analogous to the presentation of words in a free association approach. Nevertheless, because the prompting materials are uniform, it is theoretically possible to categorize and "standardize" answers, a basis for psychometrics, or mental measurement. For this reason, they are also used by non-Freudian therapists who prefer a testing approach to the primarily clinical (nonexperimental) and intuitive approach of psychoanalysis.

It would be tempting to distinguish between the production and the response approaches by suggesting that the former rest on the intuitive analysis of authentic expression, while the latter is a quantified "scientific" approach based on statistical frequency of response. Such a distinction, however, would not hold up. For one thing, virtually all of the psychometricians who have reviewed the projective tests agree that none is really a test; neither the *reliability* (consistency of measurement) nor the *validity* (the degree to which they measure what they purport to measure) of any of the projective tests has been established. They suggest hypotheses, but they do not measure.

Moreover, the attempt to quantify and to create measurement scales seems to cut across the distinction between production and response. Several investigators have tried to establish correlations between personality and the drawing of human figures based on statistical frequency of response.[19] Most such correlations focus on the placement of the figure, the presence, absence, or distortion of body features, the presence of buttons, the degree of precision in the drawing itself, and the presence or absence of facial expression. For example, Elizabeth M. Koppitz has developed the Human Figure Drawing Test (HFDT) for the measurement of children's mental and emotional development on the basis of their response to an instruction to "draw a whole person." Only one drawing is used for the test, for which Koppitz provides a scoring key for thirty *developmental items* and a number of *emotional indicators*.[20]

Most such attempts to quantify or correlate responses have provoked considerable criticism from those art therapists who deny that individuals' art products can be interpreted with any degree of precision in the absence of corroborating data. For example, while Koppitz warns against simple one-to-one interpretations,[21] critics point to her own assignment of meaning to specific features or to their absence. A slanting figure is an apparent "sign of instability and imbalance which interferes with academic achievement"[22] and suggests that the child lacks a secure footing. Tiny figures mean timidity, large figures suggest aggression, and small heads "indicate intense feelings of intellectual inadequacy."[23]

While Koppitz presumably intended that such interpretations be used as suggestive hypotheses, simple correlations have drawn the ire of critics. Referring to the approach as "blind analysis," Rhoda Kellog contends that "pictorial capacity . . . does not exist until the child is trained to substitute an adult's idea of how lines 'should be drawn' for his own highly developed and natural ideas about drawing."[24] Kellog argues, too, that any inferences about the intellectual or emotional development of a child based on a single drawing are almost inevitably distorted, because children's drawings of figures are remarkably inconsistent, even over a short span of time.

Such attempts to catalog or score responses, as in the TAT or in drawings, as in the HFDT, are not tests, no matter what they are called, according to psychometricians. Dale B. Harris of the Pennsylvania State University, reviewing the HFDT for the *Seventh Mental Measurements Yearbook*, writes:

> The HFDT is not . . . a test but an evaluation of presumptive clinical evidence. It adds little that is objective or quantifiable to the subjective or "clinical" use of drawings. . . . Depending on the psychologist's use of and belief in qualitative and subjective evidence, the HFDT may be used along with other evidence, qualitative or quantitative, to illuminate and clarify the clinical picture of personality where disturbances are known or strongly suspected.[25]

Some believe that the greatest promise for diagnosis rests on the consensus that sensitivity to color provides important clues to personality, an agreement that cuts across the production/perception barrier. A number of investigators contend that color preference is a more sensitive indicator of emotion than are form and shape; the latter apparently invite intellectual rather than emotional response.[26] Because the range of color preference can be ascertained easily and quickly, some therapists have attempted to establish a conversion scale of color response to emotional state. The Zierer Technique, for example, uses response to color as the key to the analysis and measurement of anxiety and/or aggression and "awareness of coping ability vis-a-vis conflicting contingencies."[27]

Attempts to standardize and norm responses to color have fared badly at the hands of reviewing psychometricians, as have attempts to standardize projective techniques. Professor S. G. Lee, head of the psychology department of Leicester University in England, for example, scornfully dismisses the Color Pyramid Test, which is designed to measure personality through color preference. Calling the rationale for the test "a grossly simplified system of hypothesized relationships" between colors and personality traits, he writes that "the enormous cross-cultural variations in colour symbolism are hardly mentioned," and he rejects the "prediction equations" that are offered as being beneath serious consideration. Lee continues:

> Here is a very short list, roughly sampled, from the norms given: "Considerate, cheerful, unquestioning, suspicious, conventional, egotistical, timid, 'quitting,' baffled, intelligent, brave." The inferential leaps to these from a basis of mere colour choice and use are too great to command the credulity of your reviewer.[28]

Most diagnosticians do not pretend to command any significant degree of precision in correlating color preference with personality. For example, Birren admits that his findings, derived from clinical practice, "have an empirical basis and are founded more on many years of observation than on any carefully conducted research. For the most part, emotional reactions are not easy to quantify."[29] Among his findings:

> Persons having an agreeable rapport with the outer world will like color; those given to inner rapport may not. . . . The outwardly oriented individual may appreciate color for the sake of color; those who are inwardly oriented require a semblance of realism if art forms are to appear to make "sense." . . .
>
> Manic-depressives in particular will be pleased by color and will react with considerable (and agreeable) excitement to it.
>
> In many forms of mental disturbance color is looked upon as an intruding and disturbing element. . . . Color shock of this nature, however, is seldom noted in manic-depressives.
>
> Schizophrenic types are inclined to reject color, to look upon it as something which may prove to be "catastrophic." . . .
>
> Hysterical persons may find it difficult to organize their thoughts coherently when color is an element to be considered. . . .
>
> To the psychoneurotic and psychotic, green is a great favorite. Probably it suggests escape from anxiety. . . . Blue is the color to be associated with schizophrenia.[30]

In a study of young children from three to five years of age, Alschuler and Hattwick found that the frequent use of blue or black indicated self-control and the repression of emotion, that red revealed uninhibited expression, that yellow indicated infantile traits, and that green showed a simple and uncomplicated nature.[31]

Between the spontaneous, free-association technique of the Freudians (and of many humanist therapists, as well) and the "standardized" and quantified approach of those who seek a psychometric or testing approach, a group of techniques have been developed that borrow from each. For example, a complex of activities and analyses have come to be associated with the *House-Tree-Person* (H-T-P) approach, in which an individual is asked to make a pencil drawing (achromatic) of a house, a tree, and a person. Afterward, he or she is asked to draw a house, a tree, and a person in crayons (chromatic). The analysis is based on the colors used by the individual, his or her approach to the drawing instruments, and the drawings themselves. Because the subject was suggested by the therapist, and the product is not completely spontaneous, the H-T-P approach may be seen as involving the "standard task" that is necessary in a test. On the other hand, a considerable amount of freedom is provided, so the process permits an element of free association.

An impressively large number of researchers have presented findings based on the use of H-T-P. Hammer found that "personality-constricted" individuals approach the crayons with hesitant anxiety, normal individuals do so with confidence, and psychotics "employ an almost savage pressure."[32] The average individual, Hammer found, uses from three to five colors for the house, two to three for the tree, and three to five for the person. For the inhibited individual, the range is often restricted to a single crayon, which is used as though it were a pencil. Those who have trouble exercising adequate control over their emotions, on the other hand, demonstrate an "over-expansive" use of color. Hammer remarks that "one psychotic recently indicated his inadequate control, as well as his break with conventional reality, by drawing each of the eight windows in his house a different color."[33] In his investigation, researcher John Payne found that anxious subjects tend to reinforce a color by going over it again and again, that schizophrenics and manics frequently produce inharmonious color combinations, and that mental defectives and "organics" tend to put excessively heavy pressure on the crayons.[34]

Other areas of general agreement on the use of color in the H-T-P are that the use of reds and yellows reflects spontaneity, while the use of blues or greens indicates control,[35] that black and brown are symptomatic of inhibition,[36] and that the overuse of yellow may be an expression of hostility and aggression.[37]

The propensity of the quantifiers to generalize has not gone unchallenged. Several observers have warned against misreading out of context and against overfacile diagnoses based on limited samples. Josef Albers warns against the tendency to focus on simply identifying the colors used in a drawing, rather than on the way the colors are used in the context of other colors.[38] And Irene Champernowne is alarmed at the tendency of many therapists to jump to conclusions on the basis of fragmentary clues. "These creative expressions," she says, "are so complex and subtle that only if one has participated as therapist *within* the moving, changing process for a long time should one dare to diagnose a human being."[39] In addition, she cautions against snap translations from one language to another, because the process of translation itself "is bound to bring loss or error."[40]

Such warnings point out a dilemma. Diagnosis of mental state through the analysis of art products has long been seen as a major function of art therapy. Indeed, it is so important that the suggestion has been made that a good criterion for the registration of art therapists might be diagnostic accuracy in the judgment of art products.[41] However, the warnings by Albers and Champernowne are underlined by the results of experimental studies on the diagnostic accuracy of art therapists. There seems to be no correlation between experience in art therapy (or, for that matter, experience in mental health in general) and accuracy in identifying the work of patients as contrasted with normal control subjects.[42] The investigators in one such study found the spread in diagnostic ability among art therapists disturbing, and they suggest that "diagnostic accuracy may be significantly related to professional merit."[43]

The issue is a critical one, because diagnosis is not limited to initial contact; unless a therapist can read the signs with some degree of accuracy throughout the therapy, there is no way of knowing whether the patient is improving or regressing or whether the treatment is effective. It is obvious that much more work and study are needed in this area. In the meantime, practitioners must avoid facile conclusions based on limited samples that are not corroborated by other evidence.

THE THERAPEUTIC USE OF ART

It would be highly inaccurate to suggest that the diagnostic function and therapeutic functions can be separated in clinical practice. Nevertheless, specific functions can be isolated and examined as functional constructs.

Catharsis

The term *kathartic* is generally attributed to Aristotle, who said that "art releases unconscious tensions and purges the soul."[44] The cathartic function, common to all the expressive therapies, is based on the finding that the expression of a problem or a concern provides relief. The artistic process itself is often sufficient for the working through and the release of tension; the function is not dependent on verbalization. A case described in a British journal illustrates this spontaneity: A troubled student was discouraged and "thoroughly sick of all his work," which he thought was useless and unrelated to real life. He was resistant to psychotherapy, but agreed to produce a small painting. The report concludes as follows:

> . . . after doing the picture, he felt much more calm and relaxed, and was able to continue with his work. . . . In this case one painting . . . expressed impulsively all the major stresses and problems of his life. . . . [He] was very unwilling to accept psychological interpretations, and these were never pressed upon him, but he was able to see the conflicts and relationships implied by the picture. It illustrated the use of art spontaneously in free expression of hostility and bitterness.[45]

Some argue that the artistic process itself offers channels of expression and of the release of deeply repressed emotions; numbers of observers have remarked on the relieving effect of expression alone. Irene Jakab writes that

> *without interpretation to the patient, art therapy serves as catharsis.* Many patients feel relieved of their anxiety while drawing the visual image of their "persecutor" or of their frightening nightmares and hallucinations. This feeling is close to the experience of primitive people who feel relieved by painting or modeling the image of their demons, and who believe they gain power over the enemy by modeling his statue. Art therapy done in sessions unrelated to the verbal psychotherapy is becoming a treatment tool used more and more in mental hospitals and outpatient treatment centers.[46]

Most such treatment, however, involves a combination of nonverbal and verbal approaches. Most art therapists believe that art therapy may be more effective when it is combined with verbal therapy (either with a psychotherapist or with the art therapist), even when the nonverbal function is merely cathartic. Jakab and Howard report a case in which a twelve-year-old girl who had witnessed a suicide had developed a school phobia and exhibited rage and panic when attempts were made to force her to attend school. In the hospital, she was resistant and uncooperative in verbal psychotherapy. After having drawn a picture of the suicide scene, however, she was able to talk about the event, and soon she joined the school classes in the hospital. The observers comment that

> in this case, art therapy was the most suitable method for dealing with the phobic symptoms, for it was the least threatening type of expression for the patient. It also served as catharsis. In art therapy she was able to deal

with the repressed memory which brought into focus her own aggressive feelings and the separation anxiety.[47]

Catharsis itself is a subject of disagreement among art therapists. Some think that the cathartic function is as incomplete from the point of view of therapy as it is from the point of view of art. Rudolf Arnheim asserts that from an aesthetic perspective, "the *mere* spontaneous outburst, the mere loosening up and letting go is as incomplete a performance artistically as it is humanly."[48] And from a therapeutic point of view as well, Irene Champernowne contends, the release of energy in itself is of questionable value. Energy without form, she writes, "can grow more evil, while evil in a recognizable shape can be met and dealt with in some way. The tension of the process of shaping may even foster good, but the work must be done with conscious deliberation. . . ." [49] What is unconscious, she claims, cannot be modified or educated until it is made conscious — and it is the *channeling* of the energy that provides its value. It is true that many patients are frightened by their own unbridled and undirected anger or aggression when it wells up in the course of therapy.

Therapists generally agree that catharsis alone may be a useful, but temporary, expedient. Deep-seated problems will surface again, and their treatment will require additional work.

Interpersonal Communication

Before they began to use phonetic symbols as the basis of written language, humans used pictorial symbols to give permanence to their expressions — and to convert them into communications. The search for meaning among early humans must have involved the desire to communicate that meaning to others. To those who are psychoanalytically inclined, this communication of personal interpretations and feelings, through symbolically expressed images, has its origin in the unconscious, which Naumburg calls "the constant vital reservoir from which all forms of creative expression draw their energies." [50]

It is extremely difficult to distinguish in a communication what is specifically designed to be a message and what is genuine self-revelation or expression. The artist Alfred Tunnelle commented that the artist does not see things as *they* are, but as *he* is, and Leonardo da Vinci observed that the person who draws or paints "is inclined to lend to the figures he renders his own bodily experiences, if he is not protected against this by long study."[51] To art therapists, the heart of the communication is precisely that element that is expressive and revealing; Naumburg contends that whether messages are understood by others or not, for disturbed patients they are attempts to communicate with others.[52]

By means of pictorial projection, the art therapist encourages patients to come out of themselves, to communicate with others, to deal with the world outside. Talking with a group of psychotic patients in a mental hospital, art therapist Elinor Ulman was forced to define art. "Art," she answered, "is the meeting ground of the world inside and the world outside."[53]

To some art therapists, the communication function is the most important single function in art therapy. In fact, Naumburg sees little that art therapy contributes to the therapeutic process *other* than the enlargement of communications possibilities. She thinks that artistic production is superior to verbal communication for many of the reasons that have already been discussed under the diagnostic function: it permits direct expression of dreams and fantasies, it minimizes self-censorship, it provides for the preservation of the communication, and it encourages the resolution of transference by permitting the patient to help in interpreting the product.

The art therapist's task is to recognize both the conscious and the unconscious elements in the message, What is being communicated? The process is complicated by the fact that the personal and subjective nature of interpersonal communication is not one-sided. Just as the sender of the message colors the communication with his or her own emotions as well as with paints, so the viewer perceives the product through emotionally tinted filters. How accurately can the art therapist translate — let alone interpret — an art product without the corroboration of verbal communication? On this question, opinion is divided. Some suggest that visual images alone may be the most effective dialogue between therapist and severely regressed and largely nonverbal patients.[54] Jungian analyst Irene Champernowne warns that verbalization may distort the communication between patient and therapist by introducing an intermediate language, with the attendant dangers of mistranslation and misinterpretation. She told an audience at the Royal College of Art in London that "the art form has its own validity and to translate from one language to another is bound to bring loss or error."[55]

Some wonder if the visual image alone may not be as distorted as a verbal communication alone. Psychiatrist Mardi Horowitz notes that while word meanings are relatively stable, visual symbols tend to be idiosyncratic, overdetermined, and open to misreading and multiple interpretations, and that an overreliance on graphic communication may encourage the patient to "pour out a rich fantasy life in graphic products and use the entire activity to avoid dealing in the real world with real problems."[56] Horowitz believes that this danger is so great that art production should not be the sole technique used in any treatment, but that verbalization is needed to bridge the gap between communication and cognitions belonging to the world of fantasy and those belonging to the world of reality.

It would appear that most art therapists combine verbal and nonverbal approaches in communication, sometimes with the art therapist probing for interpretation and encouraging the patient to talk about a picture, but more often with the art therapist acting in concert with a verbal psychotherapist. Irene Jakab believes there must be a two-way communication:

> The psychotherapist learns what is going on in art therapy, not only by looking at the patient's production, but by being informed by the art therapist of the patient's behavior. The art therapist has to be informed about the patient's progess and the major problems being worked through at various stages of the verbal therapy.[57]

A rapidly growing area in art therapy is focused on family relationships. Family drawings are used for communication, not only between a subject and a therapist, but between family members themselves as well. Hanna Y. Kwiatkowska, who pioneered the use of such family art therapy at the National Institute of Mental Health, found that the sessions in which all family members were involved were not only therapeutic in terms of overall family relationships, but among individual kinships as well. The family drawings, which Kwiatkowska interpreted psychoanalytically, revealed much about the relationships between family members and about the perceptions of the individuals about the role and status of each member. Kwiatkowska saw her program as a combination of spontaneous art expression and some standardized tasks that make the drawings useful in comparing perceptions. The same tasks were given to each newly admitted family. "Together," says Kwiatkowska, "these procedures give us an astonishingly clear view of all [the family's] members and their transactional systems."[58]

Family drawings have been used by psychotherapists as well as by art therapists. A major difference in approach seems to be the propensity of psychologists to categorize and score responses. One development in family drawing approaches has been the use of *kinetic*, or movement, family drawings (K-F-Ds), developed for use with children by psychologist Robert C. Burns and psychiatrist S. Harvard Kaufman. By having the subject produce a drawing in which figures are moving or doing something, they contend, they get "much more valid and dynamic material in the attempt to understand the psychopathology of children in a family setting."[59]

Burns and Kaufman use many of the diagnostic elements that are employed in akinetic, or static, drawings. Particularly, they focus on the elements suggested by Karen Machover.[60] Among these, shading or scribbling suggest preoccupation, fixation, and anxiety; emphasis on buttons suggests dependency; enlargement or exaggeration of body parts suggests a preoccupation with those parts and/or their functions; omission of body parts may indicate a denial of their functions; crosshatching suggests obsession; overprecise drawings may reflect a concern for structure or an attempt to control a threatening environment; and pressure is indicative of inner or outer direction of impulse.

In addition, Burns and Kaufman are concerned with kinetic elements: style, actions, relationships. A K-F-D analysis sheet has been developed as an aid in the diagnostic interpretation of the kinetic family drawings; it is essentially a guide in checklist form that directs attention to five basic elements:

1. *Style.* Does the subject compartmentalize? Edge the drawings? Underline individual figures?
2. *Symbols.* What traditional Freudian symbolism is present?
3. *Actions.* What are individual family members doing? What actions can be identified *between* family members?
4. *Physical characteristics.* For each individual, what characteristics are apparent in terms of arm extensions? Elevation? Which figures are in front, in back, hanging? For which members have body parts been omitted? What erasures are apparent? Which family members have been omitted entirely?
5. *K-F-D grid.* How are family members placed? What is their relative height? What are the distances between family members?

While some art therapists have adopted the kinetic family drawing approach, others resent what they see as an overstructuring in the field and an appropriation of basic art therapy techniques by psychotherapists. It is likely that the field of family art therapy will grow as a result of contributions from art therapists and psychotherapists alike.

Communicating with the Unconscious

To some groups of therapists, the art process *alone* can be healing. This view cuts across compartmentalization by psychotherapeutic theory. Although the supporting arguments may vary, Freudians and Jungians can be found in alliance with humanists on this issue.

The most clearly developed theoretical position for this view derives from Freudian theory and is probably best expressed by Edith Kramer. Kramer contends that art therapy is far more than a specialized form of psychotherapy and that its value rests on the *creative* act. She writes: "When visual symbols are used mainly to supplement the spoken word in the interchange between therapist and patient, as in the art therapy of practitioners such as Margaret Naumburg, the creative act is of secondary importance and usually remains abortive."[61] In contrast, Kramer believes that the healing potentialities of art therapy reside in "the psychological processes that are activated in creative work."[62]

At the heart of this healing is the process that Freud called *sublimation*, in which sexual energy and aggressive drives are transformed into socially acceptable forms. Sublimation involves the gratification of the artist's unconscious desires and wishes, and the release of otherwise dammed-up tension, in the process of creating a work of art. Some psychoanalysts have gone even further. According to Ghadirian:

> Rank presented a theory in which he says [the] artist stands between
> the dreamer and the neurotic, and his artistic production represents
> his struggle to free himself from internal conflicts. . . . Saks saw guilt
> as a motivating power for creativity through which the artist tries to
> free himself from the anguish of guilt.[63]

Kramer thinks that the act of creating an artistic product involves the channeling, the reduction, and the transformation of aggression and potentially dangerous energies. It is an "act of integration and synthesis which is performed by the ego, wherein the peculiar fusion between reality and fantasy, between the conscious and the unconscious, which we call art is reached."[64] The stress is on *creativity*, not merely on communication, and Kramer sees the aesthetic value of the work as an indicator of sublimation at work. She writes:

> Some kinds of therapeutic application . . . are almost of necessity inim-
> ical to art. For example, whenever pictorial expression is used primarily
> for communication in psychotherapy, it is unlikely that the product

will be art. . . . Pictorial communication in psychotherapy has served
its purpose when meaning is understood by patient and therapist. . . .
Since the artistic value of the work produced is a sign of successful sublimation, the quality of the work becomes a measure (though not the
only measure) of therapeutic success.[65]

Because artistic production represents the rechanneling of
otherwise destructive tendencies, it contributes to "temporary alleviation or partial remission of pathology."[66] But more important,
Kramer believes, the process of art production provides an opportunity to work out "equivalents" for daily life experiences. Although
art cannot directly help resolve conflict, it can serve to provide "a
model of ego functioning," a "sanctuary," where new attitudes and
feelings can be expressed and tried out. The function of producing
art as therapy is "to create a symbolic living, which allows experimentation with ideas and feelings."[67] It makes apparent the conflicts, complexities, and contradictions in life, and it demonstrates
that order can be created out of chaos. In effect, creating art is living
life in microcosm, in analogy.

The function of the art therapist, in Kramer's structure, is to
encourage creative production and to lend technical assistance
and emotional support. To do this, of course, the art therapist must
be able to recognize sublimation and never allow it to degenerate
into mere catharsis or to dissipate into play or fantasy.

For the most part, the view that art itself is healing seems
to represent a minority position among psychoanalytically inclined
art therapists. Most such therapists agree that creative production
reflects or represents a communication with the unconscious, but
few, apparently, are willing to accept a role that excludes interpretation. This position is held by Freudians and Jungians alike, although
the Jungian view rests on an expanded concept of communication
from the unconscious that actively encourages artistic production.
Irene Champernowne sees art expression and art production as the
temporary holding of the repressed elements until the therapist can
enter the process with the patient and "live through it in its fantasy
and symbolic so-called art form with the creator."[68]

Jung conceived of a dialogue between the conscious and the
unconscious in which messages travel in both directions. In its
reaction to real phenomena that come through the senses—sights,
sounds, smells, textures—the conscious mind transforms the sensations into perceptions. But some experiences go unnoticed; others
are forgotten, repressed, or otherwise lost to the conscious mind and
are stored in the personal unconscious. At a deeper level is the col-

lective unconscious, the vast collection of inherited influences from the entire human race, in which the common experiences and strivings are coagulated into archetypes, or complexes, based on accumulated and shared racial memories.

To Jung, there is much to be learned from the unconscious if individuals permit and encourage such communication, which always comes indirectly in the form of symbols. Jung saw the encouragement of the dialogue as progress toward wholeness or unity. The images and symbols must be accepted by the conscious, even when they cannot be fully understood.

Unlike Freud, Jung saw art as a valuable device with which to capture fleeting dream-images. In his autobiographical *Memories, Dreams, Reflections*, Jung mentions a dream-image that he did not understand, and so "I painted it in order to impress it upon my memory."[69]

How does an individual tune in to the unconscious? Doodling, which is often used for diagnostic purposes,[70] is seen also as a particularly valuable tool for bringing to the surface the hitherto hidden elements of the unconscious. Jacobi remarks that "the truth of the unconscious, in contrast to the conscious, position is often revealed in doodlings produced during serious conferences, and this frequently must astonish the doodler."[71] Emanuel Hammer believes that "doodles tend to tap even deeper layers of personality than do other types of drawings because doodles are usually produced in a diminished state of consciousness when the patient's focus of attention is on other matters, his control lowered, and defensiveness, which might at other times be operative, relatively put aside."[72]

To Jungian analysts, the ultimate expression of the dialogue between the conscious and the unconscious is the creation of *mandalas*, the Sanskrit word for "circles." These often ornate circle drawings are viewed as cryptograms; in Jung's own terms, they are the expression of self and the path to the center, to individuation.[73] The symbol of the circle denoting unity, and the drawing of mandalas, of course, did not originate with Jung. In fact, Jung himself stressed the ancient nature of such drawings, which he saw as archetypal. However, the impact of the mandala on the field of art therapy is generally attributed to Jung, who perceived in such images "the symbol which embraces both conscious and unconscious and unites them."[74]

The mandala has been seized upon by numbers of humanist therapists, who, like Jung, see in it a symbol of integration and unity.

Like him, they see in mandalas a form that is self-healing as well as self-revealing.[75]

Like analytical art therapists, humanists generally accept the concept of an unconscious. They, too, talk of the integration of personality (although they may not mean by the term what the Freudians mean), and they, too, see the artistic endeavors of patients, the products of such endeavors, and attempts by patients to translate and interpret their work as ways of probing the unconscious. Humanists, though, are less likely than analytical art therapists to distinguish between "normal" and "abnormal" individuals or behaviors. The humanist view of an integrated personality is more likely to be expressed in terms of self-actualization or self-fulfillment than of mental health or normality. As a result, they are likely to focus on growth rather than on understanding, on acceptance of messages from the unconscious, rather than on analysis. As a result, the line between normal self-growth and therapy is blurred. In gestalt therapy, especially, it is often not clear when writers use words in their therapy-related sense and when they use them in their perceptive-psychological sense. Here, for example, is an artist writing as an artist, not as a therapist:

> The word Gestalt, which means form, stands for our tendency to perceive visual patterns as unified configurations. Accordingly, in a Gestalt we seize a visual experience instantaneously and whole, as in a single perception. We do this because we are psychologically driven to make the experience symmetrical and complete, and this necessity in turn requires an act of closure in which each of us imposes his own order upon it.[76]

Gestalt art therapists use concepts that are strikingly similar when they talk of "integrating" experiences, of breaking barriers to wholeness. Janie Rhyne, a leader in gestalt art therapy, for example, prefers to talk of gestalt art experience rather than gestalt art therapy. She writes:

> Now I must define simply what I mean by the *gestalt art experience.* This drawing of my fantasies, I can see them, I can read my messages, I can learn; I can integrate my past childhood with my present and with visions of my future. I think of my expressive drawings as sources of learning serving me somewhat as my dreams do. These are different from the dreams I experience during sleep but alike in that both kinds of imagery can provide a path not only into the suppressed feelings of me as a child but also into present recognition of what I need and want now. They show how I, as a mature person, can bring all of these realizations together into the pattern of my own gestalt, whose every part is related to the total configuration that is me — past, present, future — and

they show that I and my environment are ever changing and ever inter-
acting.[77]

A key word in gestalt is *interrelationships*. The principles of
gestalt psychology — the need for closure, the drive toward integration and meaning — are clearly illustrated in the visual arts. The
artist's need to produce a work that has unity and form is matched
by the viewer's need to see a whole, to relate isolated parts to each
other, to see a "belonging together" of disparate elements. The
viewer who looks at an interrupted circle will complete and close the
circle in his mind's eye. A central thesis in gestalt art therapy is, in
Rhyne's words: "The way we perceive visually is directly related to
how we think and feel."[78] The patterns of art products reveal something about the pattern of the creator's life; the structure (or the lack
of it) is related to the individual's behavior in living situations. To
Rhyne, an art product is evidence of how we perceive our own lives,
and from it we can gain "new insights into how we can use our
perceptiveness to create more integrated lives."[79]

Because behaviorists question the very existence of an unconscious, the integrative function would not normally be considered a
major element in any behavior-modification program. But true
behavior modification is hard to find in art therapy. (Where it *is*
described in the literature, it often seems to bear on the "appro-
priateness" of behavior during the therapy sessions, rather than
on the art therapy functions themselves.) On the other hand, there
is evidence that some of the principles of behaviorism (and certainly a number of underlying assumptions) have found their way
into the increasingly "eclectic" practice of art therapy. In the following comments by Mihaly Csikszentmihalyi, we can find a liberal
sprinkling of terms and concepts that have been adopted from both
behaviorism and humanism:

> If we accept the proposition that emotional disturbances usually have their
> origins in frustrated existential needs, then it follows that the therapeutic
> potential of art consists in providing a symbolic [reward] system within
> which a person can develop skill and competence, and thereby obtain
> positive information about himself. This means that art . . . can give sus-
> tenance to the basic psychological need of proving one's existence. . . .
>   The purpose of art therapists should be to trick the patient into the
> use of art as a skill. If the trick works, the patient will gain a dimension of
> autonomy, a source of information which validates his being. . . .
>   Let me make clear that I am not using the verb "to trick" in a
> derogatory sense. After all, we are all tricked from birth on into accepting

the material values of our culture. Emotionally disturbed patients are tricked to believe themselves to be helpless and ineffective. It is only fair that we should use the same process to restore a positive self-concept to those who lack it.[80]

Mood Change and Sedation

Image formation and emotional state are intimately connected. Just as the emotions shape and color images, some art therapists believe, so conscious image formation can be used to change moods and attitudes.[81] The use of imagery for mood change apparently is limited in practicality. A mildly depressed individual who follows instructions to draw "a happy scene" may find that his or her outlook changes temporarily. More important, the experience may serve as a reminder that the depression itself is not a permanent state. The use of imagery for mood change is of little practical use in dealing with seriously depressed or disturbed patients; even if these patients agree to draw such "mood-change" scenes, it is more than likely that the drawing that emerges will reflect the underlying unconscious emotions and attitudes. Mood-change techniques apparently are appropriate to "normal neurotics" rather than to psychotic patients.

It is with a certain reluctance and hesitancy that sedation is proposed as a function of art therapy. There are two reasons for this reluctance: in terms of strict denotation, sedation is not properly therapeutic; and very little is found in the literature on sedation, outside of the rather obvious finding that certain colors are calming, while others may aggravate some psychoses. Faber Birren suggests that "patients in a frantic and manic state may require sedation with color, blue and green tones, dim illumination. The extremely melancholic may need a compensating warmth of hue."[82] Possibilities suggest themselves for the use of color sedation, and some art therapists may suggest the use of specific colors to patients involved in art therapy; little reference has been found, however, in the literature on the active employment of color as sedation. For the most part, color sedation seems to be limited to the obvious: painting walls and hanging drapes in calming colors in offices and hospital wards. Because psychotic patients with a variety of disorders may be found together in most hospital wards and activity rooms, even this approach seems to have limited practical value.

Color Therapy

At one end of the art therapy spectrum, as we have already seen, the discipline and practice edge over into verbal psychotherapy. At the other end, there is a seepage from practices that many art therapists reject as mystical, esoteric, and metaphysical.

A hard kernel of evidence indicates that color influences mood, that color choice may reflect aspects of personality, and that color is intimately associated with emotion. Around the edges of this evidence have grown some schools of color use that focus on the healing qualities of color and light. At the more conservative end of this movement stands Faber Birren, a color consultant who has spent years studying the psychology of color perception, the interrelation of color preference and personality, and the practical application of color for business and education.[83] At the other end is a cluster of esoteric and semireligious approaches.

Underlying the more metaphysical approaches are some principles that, interestingly enough, seem to have spun off from some solid scientific findings. One underlying concept is that of the *aura*, a luminous electromagnetic field that surrounds every living organism. Auric sight—the ability to see and analyze the aura—can be developed by long practice, but aura goggles are available to do-it-yourself practitioners—and, like so much in the newer therapies, a good deal in color healing is based on a do-it-yourself approach.[84]

While there are some differences in theory and practice among some of the color healers, most of the color therapies rest on the principle that color is a life force. A disharmony in the color vibrations of an individual is an indication of an imbalance in that individual's glandular or psychic functioning. Moreover, an individual's color preferences may be an indication of a subconscious reaching out for "healing" colors, and appropriate color therapy may involve "color baths," or "color breathing" in the pure colors in which the individual is deficient. The colors of the light rays are then transformed into revitalizing energies that charge the life centers (glands) that are debilitated.[85]

Given so wide a range in the use of color in therapy, it is not surprising that at least some elements of color healing should overlap generally accepted principles in art therapy. And such names as that of Faber Birren are acknowledged equally in the fields of art therapy and color therapy. For the most part, however, art therapists seem to be skeptical about the more unorthodox of the color-healing theories. And while some have worked with some elements of color therapy, others, including humanist art therapists, have been outspoken in their rejection of color healing as a "novelty therapy" that should not be associated with humanist art therapy.

CURRENT ISSUES IN ART THERAPY

As we have seen, the definition of art therapy adopted by the American Art Therapy Association was itself an attempt to placate divergent groups. The division that was apparently perceived at that time lay along the lines of psychotherapeutic affiliation or preference. However, the fundamental differences that have become increasingly apparent go far deeper; they focus on the relative stress on *art or therapy* in art therapy. Accordingly, art therapists tend to see their work either as *art in therapy* or *art as therapy*.

We have touched on this disagreement in dealing with the functions of communication and integration. Art therapy pioneer Margaret Naumburg sees the primary value of art therapy in authentic expression and in communication, in which the images produced by the patient are a form of symbolic speech. Naumburg is skeptical about claims that the process of art production itself has any special healing value.

At the other end of this argument stands another art therapy pioneer, Edith Kramer, who shares with Naumburg an analytical bias. Kramer thinks that art is itself healing. In her view, the creative act is an act of sublimation—of channeling, reducing, and transforming potentially destructive or antisocial energies. It is an act of personality integration. Moreover, artistic production provides for working with "equivalents" and analogues. In the artistic act, conflict is reexperienced, resolved, and integrated. The art therapist's major goal is to help the patient *express* conflicts, not *interpret*, them.

Describing the schism, Elinor Ulman writes that in terms of Naumburg's definitions, "Kramer is an art teacher rather than an art therapist. Into Kramer's ideological scheme, Naumburg fits as a psychotherapist, not an art therapist."[86] Admittedly, as Ulman points out, this is an extreme statement of the cleavage "between those art therapists who operate near the peripheral area of psychotherapy at the one side, and those who operate near the peripheral area of art education at the other."[87] Ulman is at some pains to explain that the disagreement in practice is not as absolute as it would appear in theory, even for such strong personalities as Naumburg and Kramer. And in practice, few analytical art therapists are so dogmatic as to exclude from their work either view. The specifics of methodology seem to be influenced more by the nature of the institution, the types of patients involved, and the specific goals at which they aim than by purely theoretical considerations.

The stress throughout this chapter has been on the psycho-analytic practice of art therapy. The reason is simple: most art therapists in this country—whether the stress is on the art or the therapy—subscribe to Freudian or neo-Freudian theories. Given the domination of the institutions of mental health by psychiatrists, it is not surprising that the functions assigned to art therapists have been largely adjunctive, primarily for diagnosis and—to a smaller degree—for catharsis. The underlying assumption seems to be that the corrective (curative-therapeutic) work is to remain the province of the (verbal) psychoanalyst-psychiatrist.

In fact, the implications of the art *in* therapy stance have not been lost on many psychiatrists who are interested in using art as an adjunct. Some contend that if creativity is not the focus of art therapy, then they are in a better position than art therapists to interpret the visual communications of their patients. *Any* attempt at interpretation, argue such medical therapists, should be left exclusively to the expert psychiatrist.[88] Such a view, obviously, would relegate art therapists to a distinctly inferior position in the hierarchies of the mental health empire. The drive toward profession-alization, discussed in some depth in Chapter 6, must inevitably be affected by the view of art therapy that prevails among psychiatrists and psychotherapists.

On philosophical grounds, the art in therapy position is vigor-ously rejected by humanists. The Naumburg view puts art therapists in the business of pseudopsychiatry, characterized, in the words of Mary Lee Hodnett, by "too much Freudian verbiage, too much un-substantiated opinion, too little art. . . ." Art therapists, she claims, are frequently—and scornfully—branded "junior psychiatrists."[89] To humanist practitioners, the psychoanalytic bias in art therapy puts art therapists in the danger of being swallowed by psychiatrists; either their functions will be taken over by psychiatrists themselves, or they will remain in the mental health field as lackeys.

The psychiatric domination, in fact, has spilled over from the hospitals and the outpatient clinics into the very bastions of art edu-cation. Art psychologist Rudolf Arnheim deplores what he calls the "psychiatric bias" that, in his view, has contaminated art education. Many teachers, he asserts, have come to realize that art is an instru-ment of human personality. But, he argues, too many such educators have fallen under the influence of the psychiatric preoccupation with abnormality; they define personality as "the manifestation of what is wrong with people, . . . [so] they scrutinize the work of their young students for signs of hostility, depression, anxiety, jealousy, and they have surprisingly little trouble in finding them. . . . One would learn very little about the solar system by concentrating on eclipses of the sun or the moon."[90]

To humanists, who see their work in terms of education at least as much as therapy, the psychoanalytic domination is a double threat. Much of the humanist effort is directed toward an attack on the traditional medical model of therapy. "My argument," contends Csikszentmihalyi, "is that the whole of society needs art therapy, not only the emotionally disturbed."[91]

The function of art, to the humanists, is basically to help each individual move toward self-actualization, or individuation, or fulfillment, or wholeness, depending on the humanist model to which the proponent subscribes. Mary Lee Hodnett concludes an argument for art therapy as a system of personality support rather than of treatment for the ill, by pleading:

> A broader view of art therapy is our plea, to stop being bound only by the concepts and interpretations of psychoanalytic theory and to move into a higher, self-actualizing level of approach, i.e., into the potential of creativity as the agent of change in restoring and maintaining mental health.[92]

While many in the field of art therapy welcome the newer and freer approaches that characterize the human potential movement, many more are uncomfortable. Like their counterparts in dance/movement therapy, many art therapists—including humanists—are often painfully aware of a danger to their discipline from the novelty therapies—often mystical and antiintellectual—that have proliferated during the 1960s and 1970s. Many of the newer semireligious therapies have borrowed indiscriminately from the expressive arts therapies and have often used these techniques for purposes that are considered questionable by leaders in these therapies.

Humanist art therapists are particularly disturbed because the novelty therapies are often popularly associated with humanism. During a symposium on divergent views in art therapy, Janie Rhyne said:

> The big umbrella of the human-potential movement—the third force in psychology—shelters a lot of diversity: existentialists, phenomenologists, mystics, Eastern philosophers—many views of the human venture. Among these is a gestalt philosophy and mode of therapy. Gestalt at its best fosters creative change and especially clear awareness of responsibilities. At its worst gestalt therapy is used as a catchall for a mishmash of "if-it-feels-good-do-it" messing around. This kind of sensation-seeking therapy is often presumed to be the norm in California.

I come from California. . . . Sometimes I feel really loaded down, being asked to justify all the kooky things people do when they get together in groups and throw paint around . . . in the name of art experience.[93]

Hodnett, also a humanist art therapist, predicts (perhaps "hopes" would be more accurate) that "many of these [novelty therapies] will fall by the wayside, dying from loss of their novelty or from weirdness and consequent failure to attract new adherents."[94]

An increasingly heard assertion, still a minority position, is the contention that art therapy is an independent discipline, not the handmaiden of any of the psychotherapies. At the general session of the Fifth Annual Convention of the American Art Therapy Association, held in New York City in 1974, Bernard I. Levy told the assembled members that "art therapy must develop its own body of knowledge expressed in its own literature if the profession is to expand and to achieve a sense of its own identity."[95]

REFERENCE NOTES

1. G. G. Thompson, *Child Psychology* (Boston: Houghton Mifflin, 1952), pp. 211-12.
2. Jean Piaget, *The Language and Thought of the Child* (New York: Meridian Books, 1955); Herbert Ginsburg and Sylvia Opper, *Piaget's Theory of Intellectual Development* (Englewood Cliffs, N.J.: Prentice-Hall, 1969); Jerome S. Bruner, R. R. Oliver, P. H. Greenfield, et al., *Studies in Cognitive Growth* (New York: John Wiley & Sons, 1966).
3. Rudolf Arnheim, *Visual Thinking* (Berkeley: University of California Press, 1969).
4. Rudolf Arnheim, *Toward a Psychology of Art* (Berkeley: University of California Press, 1966).
5. American Art Therapy Association, *Directory*, 1977-1978, p. 1.
6. Edith Wallace, "Art Therapists in Search of Identity: An Attempt to Define," American Art Therapy Association, *Creativity in the Art Therapist's Identity*, Proceedings, Seventh Annual Conference 1977, p. 89.
7. Sigmund Freud, *The Psychopathology of Everyday Life*, trans. A. A. Brill (London: Ernest Benn, 1935), p. 63.
8. Sigmund Freud, *New Introductory Lectures in Psychoanalysis*, Part II, ed. and trans. J. Strachey (London: The Hogarth Press, 1963), p. 90.
9. Margaret Naumburg, *Dynamically Oriented Art Therapy: Its Principles and Practices* (New York: Grune and Stratton, 1966), p. 2.

10. A. M. Ghadirian, "Artistic Expression of Psychopathology Through the Media of Art Therapy," *Confinia Psychiat.* 17 (1974):162-70.
11. Mardi J. Horowitz, "The Use of Graphic Images in Psychotherapy," *American Journal of Art Therapy* 10, no. 3 (April 1971):156.
12. Jolande Jacobi, "Compulsive Symptoms in Pictures from the Unconscious," in *Conscious and Unconscious Expressive Art Theories, Methodology and Pathographies*, ed. Irene Jakab, *Proceedings*, Fourth Annual Meeting of the American Society of Psychopathology of Expression (Basel: S. Karger, AG, 1971), pp. 103-04.
13. Naumburg, *Dynamically Oriented Art Therapy*, pp. 8-9.
14. Emery I. Gondor, *Art and Play Therapy* (Garden City, N.Y.: Doubleday, 1954), p. 29.
15. Paul Jay Fink, "Art as a Reflection of Mental Status," *Art Psychotherapy* 1 (1973):19.
16. Janie Rhyne, *The Gestalt Art Experience* (Belmont, Calif.: Wadsworth, 1973), p. 242.
17. "Symposium: Integration of Divergent Points of View in Art Therapy," *American Journal of Art Therapy* 14, no. 1 (October 1974):13.
18. Oscar K. Buros, ed., *Seventh Mental Measurements Yearbook*, 1972; *Eighth Mental Measurements Yearbook*, 1978 (Highland Park, N.J.: Gryphon Press).
19. Karen Machover, *Personality Projection in the Drawing of the Human Figure* (Springfield, Ill.: Charles C Thomas, 1949); R. C. Burns and S. H. Kaufman, *Kinetic Family Drawings* (New York: Brunner/Mazel, 1970); M. Shildkrout, I. R. Shenker, and Marsha Sonnenblick, *Human Figure Drawing in Adolescence* (New York: Brunner/Mazel, 1972).
20. Elizabeth M. Koppitz, *Psychological Evaluation of Children's Figure Drawings* (New York: Grune and Stratton, 1968), p. 55.
21. Ibid., p. 58.
22. Ibid., p. 52.
23. Ibid., p. 61.
24. Rhoda Kellog, *Analyzing Children's Art* (Palo Alto, Calif.: National Press Books, 1970), p. 189.
25. Buros, *Seventh Mental Measurements Yearbook*, p. 413.
26. David Katz, *Gestalt Psychology* (New York: Ronald Press, 1950).
27. American Art Therapy Association, *Proceedings*, 1977, p. 66.
28. Buros, *Seventh Mental Measurements Yearbook*, p. 398.
29. Faber Birren, "Color Preferences as a Clue to Personality," *Art Psychotherapy* 1 (1973):14.
30. Ibid., pp. 14-15.
31. Rose H. Alschuler and La Berta W. Hattwick, *Painting and Personality* (Chicago: University of Chicago Press, 1947).
32. Emanuel F. Hammer, "The Chromatic H-T-P, a Deeper Personality-Tapping Technique," in *The Clinical Application of Projective Drawings*, ed. E. F. Hammer (Springfield, Ill.: Charles C Thomas, 1958), pp. 231-32.

33. Ibid., p. 232.
34. John J. Payne, "Comments on the Analysis of Chromatic Drawings," in *The H-T-P Techniques: A Quantitative and Qualitative Scoring Manual,* ed. J. N. Buck, *Clinical Psychol. Monogr.* 5 (1948):1–120.
35. J. Zimmerman and L. Garfinkel, "Preliminary Study of the Art Productions of the Adult Psychotic," *Psychiatric Quarterly* 16 (1942).
36. I. Bieber, "Art in Psychotherapy," *American Journal of Psychiatry* 104 (1948).
37. M. Brick, "The Mental Hygiene Value of Children's Art Work," *American Journal of Orthopsychiatry* 14 (1944).
38. Josef Albers, *Interaction of Color* (New Haven:Yale University Press, 1975), pp. 8–9, 18–19, 22–23, 33.
39. H. Irene Champernowne, "Art and Therapy: An Uneasy Partnership," *American Journal of Art Therapy* 10, no. 3 (April 1971):141.
40. Ibid.
41. Elinor Ulman and Bernard I. Levy, "Art Therapists as Diagnosticians," *American Journal of Art Therapy* 13, no. 1 (October 1973), 37.
42. Ibid., pp. 35–38.
43. Ibid., p. 37.
44. Ernst Kris, *Psychoanalytic Explorations in Art* (New York: International Universities Press, 1952), p. 45.
45. R. W. Pickford, "Aspects of Art Therapy," *British Journal of Psychology and Personality Study* 19, no. 1 (June 1974):17.
46. Irene Jakab, "Coordination of Verbal Psychotherapy and Art Therapy," *Psychiatry and Art* 2 (1966):95.
47. Irene Jakab and M. C. Howard, "Art Therapy With a 12-Year Old Girl Who Witnessed a Suicide and Developed School Phobia," *Psychother., Psychosom.* 17 (1969):323.
48. Quoted in Champernowne, "Art and Therapy: An Uneasy Partnership," p. 139.
49. Ibid.
50. Margaret Naumburg, "Spontaneous Art in Education and Psychotherapy," in *Art Therapy in Theory and Practice,* eds. Elinor Ulman and Penny Dachinger (New York: Schocken Books, 1975), p. 221.
51. Emanuel F. Hammer, "Projection in the Art Studio," in Hammer, *The Clinical Application of Projective Drawings,* p. 8.
52. Naumburg, *Dynamically Oriented Art Therapy,* p. 45.
53. Elinor Ulman, "Therapy Is Not Enough," in Ulman and Dachinger, *Art Therapy in Theory and Practice,* p. 21.
54. Yoshihito Tokuda, "Image and Art Therapy," *Art Psychotherapy* 1 (1973).
55. Champernowne, "Art and Therapy: An Uneasy Partnership," pp. 141–42.
56. Horowitz, "The Use of Graphic Images in Psychotherapy," p. 159.
57. Jakab, "Coordination of Verbal Psychotherapy and Art Therapy," p. 97.
58. Hanna Y. Kwiatkowska, "Family Art Therapy and Family Art Evaluations," in *Proceedings,* Fourth Annual Meeting of the American Society of Psychopathology of Expression, 1971, p. 139.

59. Robert C. Burns and S. Harvard Kaufman, *Kinetic Family Drawings (K-F-D)* (New York: Brunner/Mazel, 1970), p. 18.
60. Machover, *Personality Projection in the Drawing of the Human Figure.*
61. Edith Kramer, *Art as Therapy with Children* (New York: Schocken Books, 1971), p. 25.
62. Ibid.
63. Ghadirian, "Artistic Expression of Psychopathology Through the Media of Art Therapy," p. 163.
64. Edith Kramer, *Art Therapy in a Children's Community* (Springfield, Ill.: Charles C Thomas, 1958), p. 23.
65. Kramer, *Art as Therapy with Children,* pp. 222-23.
66. Ibid., p. 207.
67. Ibid., p. 219.
68. Champernowne, "Art and Therapy: An Uneasy Partnership," p. 134.
69. Carl G. Jung, *Memories, Dreams, Reflections,* trans. Richard and Clara Winston, ed. Aniela Jaffé (New York: Random House, Vintage Books, 1965), p. 183.
70. Emanuel F. Hammer, "Doodles: An Informal Projective Technique," in Hammer, *The Clinical Application of Projective Drawings,* pp. 135-61.
71. Ibid., p. 562.
72. Ibid., p. 582.
73. Carl G. Jung, *Man and His Symbols* (Garden City, N.Y.: Doubleday, Windfall, 1964), p. 196.
74. Quoted in Champernowne, "Creative Expression and Ultimate Values," *American Journal of Art Therapy* 16, no. 1 (October 1976):6.
75. M. F. Keyes, *The Inward Journey: Art as Psychotherapy for You* (Millbrae, Calif.: Celestial Arts, 1974), pp. 59-63.
76. W. C. Libby, *Color and the Structural Sense* (Englewood Cliffs, N.J.: Prentice-Hall, 1974), p. 104.
77. Rhyne, *The Gestalt Art Experience,* p. 239.
78. Ibid., p. 242.
79. Ibid.
80. Mihaly Csikszentmihalyi, "The Release of Symbolic Energy," American Art Therapy Association, *Proceedings* (1977):100-01.
81. Horowitz, "The Use of Graphic Images in Psychotherapy," p. 159.
82. Birren, "Color Preference as a Clue to Personality," p. 15.
83. Birren, *Color—A Survey in Words and Pictures* (New York: Universe Books, 1963); *Color in Your World* (New York: Macmillan, 1962); *Color Psychology and Therapy* (New York: Universe Books, 1961); *Principles of Color* (New York: Van Nostrand Reinhold, 1969).
84. W. J. Colville, *The Human Aura and the Significance of Color* (Mokelume Hill, Calif.: Health Research, 1976); W. E. Butler, *How to Read the Aura* (New York: Samuel Weiser, 1971); Anonymous, *The Aura and What It Means to You,* a compilation of writings (Mokelume Hill, Calif.: Health Research, 1955); Oscar Bagnall, *The Origin and Properties of the Human Aura* (New York: Samuel Weiser, 1970).

85. Mary Anderson, *Colour Healing* (New York: Samuel Weiser, 1975); Anonymous, *Color Healing* (Mokelume Hill, Calif.: Health Research, 1956); Linda Clark, *Color Therapy* (Old Greenwich, Conn.: Devin-Adair, 1975); Linda Clark and Yvonne Martine, *Health, Youth and Beauty Through Color Breathing* (Millbrae, Calif.: Celestial Arts, 1976).
86. Elinor Ulman, "Art Therapy: Problems of Definition," Ulman and Dachinger, in *Art Therapy in Theory and Practice*, p. 10.
87. Ibid., pp. 10–11.
88. Ibid., pp. 4–5.
89. Mary Lee Hodnett, "Toward Professionalization of Art Therapy: Defining the Field," *American Journal of Art Therapy* 12, no. 2 (January 1973): 110.
90. Arnheim, *Toward a Psychology of Art*, p. 338.
91. Csikszentmihalyi, "The Release of Symbolic Energy," p. 100.
92. Mary Lee Hodnett, "A Broader View of Art Therapy," *Art Psychotherapy* 1 (1973):79.
93. "Symposium: Integration of Divergent Points of View in Art Therapy," p. 15.
94. Hodnett, "Toward Professionalization of Art Therapy," p. 111.
95. "Symposium: Integration of Divergent Points of View in Art Therapy," p. 13.

THE THEMATIC APPERCEPTION TEST

Developed in 1935, the TAT is designed, in the words of its creator, Henry H. Murray, to reveal to the trained interpreter "some of the dominant drives, emotions, sentiments, complexes, and conflicts of a personality."

The test consists of twenty cards that show scenes involving people. The subject is shown the cards one at a time and is asked to make up a complete story for each, describing the events that have led up to the scene, as well as the characters' actions, feelings, thoughts, and motives, and the outcome of the story. The therapist analyzes the subject's interpretation, in light of his or her personal knowledge of the subject, but considers the *content* of the stories (plot, characters, etc.) and the *form*, or the way the story was told. The therapist-interviewer looks for clues in the answers to such questions as:

1. Did the subject identify with the hero or heroine?
2. What did the attitudes of the characters reveal about the subject?
3. What contextual clues can be found in content, language, organization, consistency, originality?
4. What recurrent themes can be found in the stories?
5. What wishes, fears, and memories emerge from the stories that the subject might not ordinarily reveal?

The disclosures usually are interpreted psychoanalytically, although the TAT is also used by nonanalytic therapists. After almost fifty years of use, psychologists still widely disagree on whether the TAT is a "test" or an "interview" because of its questionable reliability (consistency) and validity (degree to which it measures what it purports to measure). The results of the studies can best be described as equivocal. Murray himself apparently did not intend, despite its title, that the TAT be used as a diagnostic *test*. He wrote in 1943 that "a blind analysis is a stunt which . . . has no place in clinical practice." The chief use of the TAT in current practice seems to be in the development of diagnostic hypotheses, to be tested by case history data and other methods.

THE RORSCHACH TEST

The Rorschach Test, also known as the Rorschach Method, the Rorschach Inkblot Test, and Rorschach Psychodiagnostics, is named after its creator, Swiss psychiatrist Hermann Rorschach, who concluded that there is a correlation between an individual's personality and the way he or she perceives form and color. Rorschach saw his "experiment" (apparently, he did not call it a test) as a standard task in which many aspects of personality could be engaged: cognitive, emotional, perceptual, social.

Each of the ten inkblots in the series, similar to those shown below, is printed on a separate card and has unique qualities of color, form, shading, and space use. Five blots are in tones of black and gray, two include red areas, and three have combinations of several colors. The cards are usually presented one at a

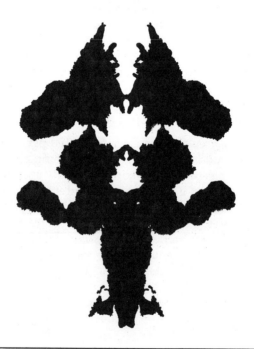

time and in a definite order. The subject is asked merely to describe what he or she sees in each card. Responses are usually scored in terms of the following criteria:

1. *Inclusiveness:* Did the response deal with the entire inkblot, or just part of it?
2. *Content:* Did the subject see a human? An animal? An inanimate object? A sexual symbol?
3. *Originality:* Was the response predictable? If original, was it linked to reality, or was it bizarre?
4. *Form:* How precise was the response? Was the concept itself simple or complex? Was it cohesive or fragmented?
5. *Properties:* What qualities were perceived: color? shape? shading? movement?

Rorschach discovered over the years that most normal individuals respond first to the whole figure, then move on to details, usually from the larger to the smaller ones. He interpreted a consistent reversal of this pattern as an indication of abnormality. So is a focus on the empty spaces in the pattern. However, Rorschach recognized that an individual who responds to all ten images with a perfectly normal reading might be displaying compulsive tendencies; most "normal" responses, he found, are symmetrical (well balanced) and not perfectly consistent. Depressed subjects are overly concerned with clear form, and their answers are stereotyped.

In particular, Rorschach saw color perception as a clue to emotional control: the withdrawn person will disregard color, a depressed person will focus on the blacks and grays, and an impulsive subject will respond in an uncontrolled, diffused way. One card, in a combination of gray, blue-green, pink, and orange-brown colors, causes "color-shock" in neurotics.

The ten images used today are those that Rorschach himself selected after years of experimentation, but the way the inkblots are used has changed considerably since 1921, when they were first published. The Rorschach originally was used as a visual free-association technique and interpreted qualitatively by the clinician. Over the years, responses have been quantified, and scoring indexes are published for use by those who administer the Rorschach as a "test."

It is generally conceded that the Rorschach is "culture biased," when used as a test. For one thing, an individual's perception is heavily influenced by his or her cultural background, as it is in body language (see Chapter 5). Primitive desert Moroccans tend to concentrate on tiny, scarcely perceptible details, while Samoans ignore details altogether, seeing only a general form, such as a bird or a fish.

Lauded and condemned, the Rorschach is one of the most reviewed, researched, and analyzed techniques extant. Charles C. McArthur of Harvard, reviewing it in the *Seventh Mental Measurements Yearbook*, calls it "a slice of total behavior [and] the only game in town" by which to discover the idiosyncratic laws of personal experience. On the other hand, others have called it unsophisticated, in terms of both measurement and personality theory.

Virtually all reviewers agree that it is too weak in inter-reader *reliability*, or consistency, to be called a test; like the blind men examining the elephant, various interpreters are looking for different things. McArthur calls the Rorschach "the richest behavior sample we know how to collect," but, he comments:

> The Rorschach is not a "test" in the sense of "tests and measures." It is a behavior sample — a standardized sample, however. . . . Paradoxically, a literature has grown up around the "psychometrics" of this nontest. . . . The Rorschach is *not* psychoanalytical [despite] recent distortions by those who "interpret" only content. . . . The Rorschach is *not* a projective test. The projective mechanism occurs in only one kind of response. Above all, it is not psychometric, nor even a measure. . . . Labelling the Rorschach as "The Rorschach Test". . . has thus erected for the delight of the captious a straw man easy to knock down.

Most psychologists see value in the Rorschach as one instrument in diagnosis. Increasingly, they are coming to view it as a "structured clinical interview" and a research tool, rather than a diagnostic measurement.

A FAMILY COPES WITH DEATH

R, nineteen years old, was dying of cancer, a disease whose course inevitably involves the readjustment of relationships within a family. R, his parents — Mr. and Mrs. M — and D, his twenty-three-year-old sister, were referred to Myra Levick, an art psychotherapist and a trained family therapist who directs the creative arts in therapy program at Hahnemann Medical College in Philadelphia.

For eight months, the family came for therapy with Levick and Morris Schimmel, then a resident in psychiatry at Hahnemann. One brother was unable to attend the sessions. In the course of art therapy, the focus was on relationships within the family and on the strain put on these relationships by R's illness and subsequent death. In fact, it was R himself who recognized his parents' and brother's inability to deal directly with his illness and with his sister's suffering; it was R who had persuaded the others to accept therapy as a family.

The first meeting was devoted to an art therapy evaluation; members of the family were asked to create a series of drawings that were subsequently discussed. A major purpose of these drawings was to have the family members recognize how much their drawings revealed of their feelings about themselves and about the other family members. After the early sessions, reported Levick, they "were marvelous to work with."

During an early family discussion, the issue arose of R's feelings after he began bimonthly chemotherapy treatments. R himself had made it clear, both at home and in the sessions, that he wanted to be left alone, and he drew himself lying sick, amid paraphernalia of illness — tissues, trash bag, etc. In her drawing, Mrs. M showed a virtually headless R lying on a couch in a position strongly suggestive of a corpse in a coffin.

During one of the sessions, it was disclosed that D had considerable anxiety about sexual relationships — an issue that was to become the focus of many later sessions, especially after R died. When the death occurred about two months after the sessions had begun, the family called and asked to

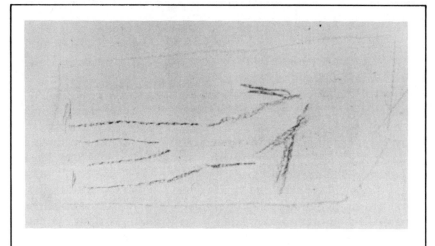

continue therapy, largely in order to cope with the changing relationship between D and her parents.

During one session, after Levick asked D to draw herself, D portrayed herself as a tree that was being observed by her parents. During her discussion of the drawing, D said that she wanted her parents to draw themselves either watering the tree or cutting it down—apparently expressing her deep-seated dependence on her parents and her need for their approval.

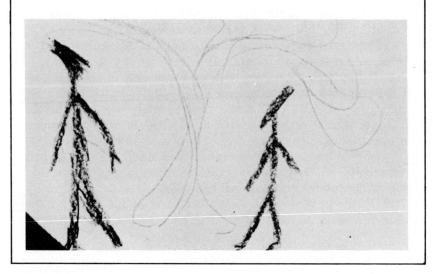

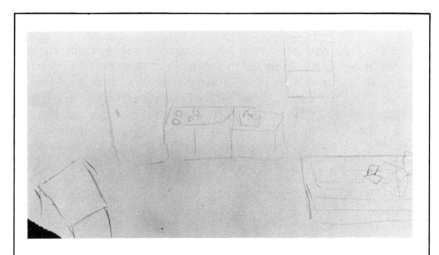

During the same general period, the family drew pictures that dealt with a recent illness suffered by Mrs. M, who expressed considerable surprise at the deep concern for her that emerged in the drawings; nobody had been able to tell her in words.

About four months after R's death, D arranged for an apartment of her own. During the session at which this move was discussed, Mrs. M drew D lying on a couch in her apartment. When Levick brought out the drawing that Mrs. M had

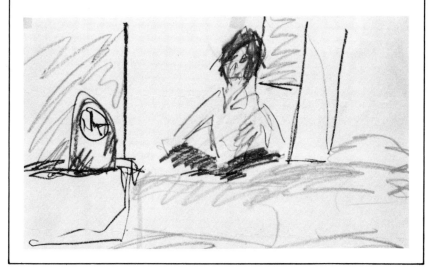

made of her son months earlier (see page 94, top), the mother realized that she perceived her daughter's move in the same terms as her son's illness, as an approaching loss. In rather sharp contrast, D drew herself with strong strokes, sitting in bed. Again, the contrast with her earlier drawing of herself as a tree suggested her newfound sense of freedom and independence.

About a month after D's move, the family terminated the sessions. "I saw the daughter in town in June," the therapist commented, "and she told me that her parents had gone to Europe and that it was the first trip they had ever taken without the children. D was very happy, working and going to law school."

Text and illustrations adapted from unpublished case notes prepared by Myra Levick, M.Ed., A.T.R., professor and director of Creative Arts in Therapy Program, Hahnemann Medical College and Hospital, Philadelphia, Pennsylvania.

SUSAN FACES HER FEARS

Ten-year-old Susan D was referred to child psychologist Hella Moller because, although she loved to read, she had difficulties adjusting to school and did poorly, especially in mathematics. According to Mr. and Mrs. D, Susan had difficulty adjusting to "almost everything," was overly rebellious, socially withdrawn, and had no girlfriends.

In addition to conducting interviews with the parents and with Susan's public school teacher, Dr. Moller administered a battery of diagnostic and personality tests, including the Wechsler Intelligence Scale for Children (WISC), the Moller Sentence Completion Test, and a wide variety of visual tests: the Draw-a-Family Test, the Bender Visual Gestalt Test, the Graham Kendal Memory for Design Test, the TAT, and the Rorschach. In addition, she relied heavily on the Kinetic Family Drawing technique. Moller believes strongly that each test or

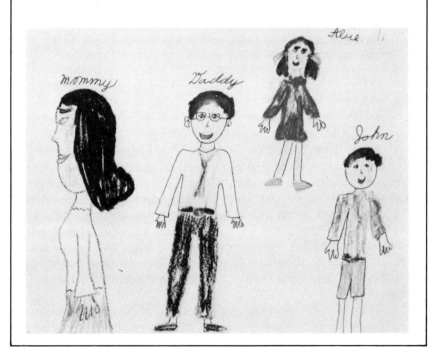

technique adds a dimension to her understanding of the child and the family relationship.

The interviews revealed that Mr. and Mrs. D were highly critical of Susan and that Mr. D's attempts to teach Susan mathematics had been highly frustrating for him and for Susan. Susan's IQ score was in the bright-normal range, but the arithmetic and coding scores on the WISC were low; this raised the question of whether Susan's basic school problem was perceptual or emotional. "Coding is an indicator of both visual motor ability and of ego strength," says Moller. On the basis of a number of other tests, Moller concluded that the problem had a basis in a "visual memory defect," possibly of organic origin, but that it was complicated by emotional aspects. In addition, Susan showed signs of "overdependency" and a need to be punished for her transgressions or deficiencies.

Susan's family drawings were revealing. Reports Moller:

> She drew her mother first, thereby indicating that she is the most important family member to her, since she was the first person that came to her mind. It is noteworthy, however, that Father, Sister, Brother and Self are drawn in front view, whereas Mother is drawn in profile, looking away from everybody as if avoiding close contact. Mother's face is nearly twice the size of the others, implying that what *she* thinks is most important to Susan. Her mouth is strong and determined. . . . The arms are rigidly pressed to the side of the body. . . . The "cut-off" in the skirt area is likely to be an indicator of some sexual anxiety in Susan regarding growing up female. In any case, Mother is not perceived as a securely grounded person.

Susan drew herself on a separate sheet of paper, suggesting to Moller that she did not relate well to her family. While the body contours were avoided, a common phenomenon among preadolescents, her hands were carefully drawn, suggesting that Susan's interest in art made her hands especially important to her. Despite Susan's use of a full vertical page for herself, her feet and part of her legs were cut off. "Unconsciously, she also shows her lack of secure footing just like Mother," remarks Dr. Moller, "and both seem to suffer from their poor relationships."

The Moller Sentence Completion suggested emotional conflict, especially between Susan and her mother, who never

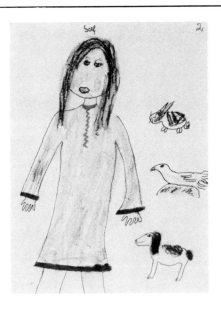

seemed satisfied with Susan. The following statements in quotes are some of her completions:

> *Mary felt that her mother* . . . "was unfair."
>
> *If I would only* . . . "have a chance to explain to my mother about things that have gone wrong."
>
> *I wish my mother* . . . "would let me bring friends home to the barn."
>
> *The worst thing that ever happened* . . . "I got in trouble and my mother would not let me explain."
>
> *I remember a dream about* . . . "a really scary dream about Mommy. Her head came off, but I am far, far away and can't find my way home."

The sentence completions relating to school showed considerable discomfort:

> *Judy felt that her teachers* . . . "were asking her impossible questions."
>
> *It is embarrassing* . . . "when people are watching and I can't do it right."
>
> *Judy worries most about* . . . "her poor school habits."

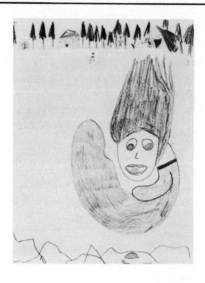

Susan's perception of herself as unreasonable and in need of punishment was corroborated by her responses to the TAT, as well as the sentence completions. The Rorschach indicated that Susan was a "passive but highly emotional girl, who has a need to deny her true feelings because she has been taught to do so. . . . Susan is at a loss in knowing how to handle her feelings, since she has been trained to repress them to a degree not appropriate for her age."

Among the recommendations in her diagnostic report: counseling for Mr. and Mrs. D to help them be more relaxed with Susan; special tutoring in a math learning disability workshop at a nearby college; and participation by Susan in Art/Interview Therapy to relieve her anxieties, help her gain more self-respect, and learn to relate warmly to a permissive adult. She also suggested that, until Susan's arithmetic improved, she not attend a regular arithmetic class "because she would be too embarrassed by her own inability."

Following the assessment, Susan participated in a combination Art/Interview Therapy program for about a year and a half. Moller asked the parents to participate in counseling because "therapy for a child cannot be effective without involvement of the family."

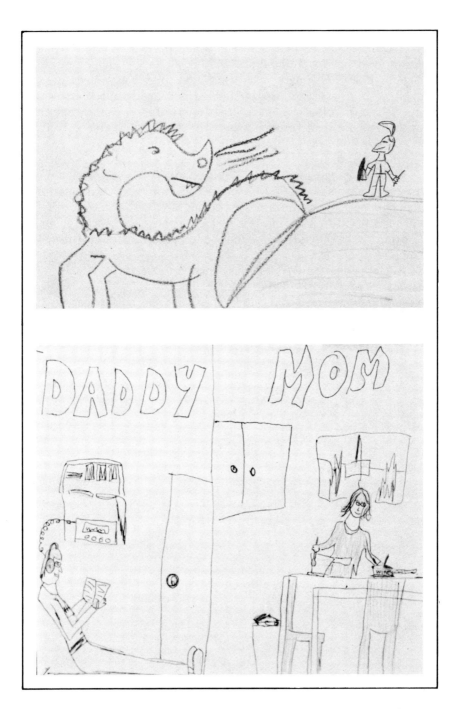

During the sessions, Susan "opened up to her therapist and relived her fears of failure and her anxiety." She expressed angers, hostilities, and fears that had previously been suppressed. In one dream, Susan showed her anguish and terror as she fell into an abyss, in a situation related to her rejection by other girls in a summer camp. In another, Father appears as a dragon who gets furious when Susan does not understand her mathematics.

"With a person's growth and change," says Moller, "the drawings also change. To promote the therapeutic progress of a person it is sometimes useful to employ verbalization—that means interpreting the meaning of the drawing with the client; at other times they are self-evident and cathartic and no [other] language is needed."

The final family drawings show considerable change in Susan's perception of her father and mother. Mother, for example, is warmer and more maternal; she cooks and cares for the family, and she looks straight ahead, no longer avoid-

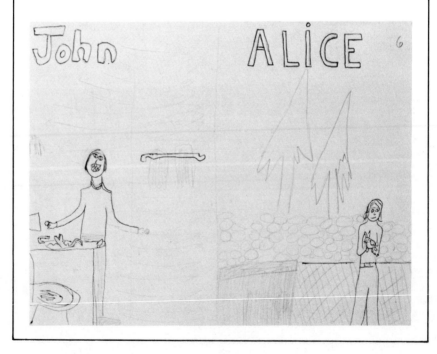

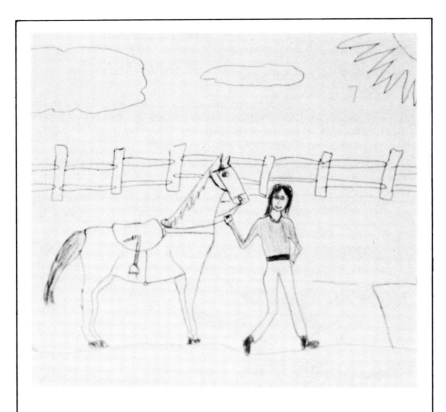

ing Susan's problems. Susan, still alone on a page, is "a whole person, striding hopefully into the world, leading her horse. Her school performance has greatly improved in a private school with more individual attention. . . . She has learned to play the guitar and has become popular with her peers."

Dr. Moller concludes:

> For Susan, Art-Interview Therapy has provided an opportunity for her to confront her fears pictorially, and make it possible to view them as figments of her imagination. She learned to cope actively with her anxiety. . . . A caring and supportive environment — in school, at home, and with her therapist — helped her to view her "inside" fears and her "outside" enemies in a more objective fashion. . . .

Abridged and adapted from an unpublished case history prepared by Hella Moller, Ed.D., Child Psychologist, Sarasota, Florida.

LORI FINDS HERSELF

Lori came with her parents and her older sister to the Thalians Community Mental Health Center of the Cedars-Sinai Medical Center in Los Angeles. Her mother, a chronic schizophrenic, had a history of numerous hospitalizations; her father was quiet and showed little emotion. Lori's sister, Frances, was seventeen, a beautiful, slender, outgoing adolescent. Lori, on the other hand, was fourteen, heavy, and clean, but disheveled, with limp hair. The initial interviewer de-

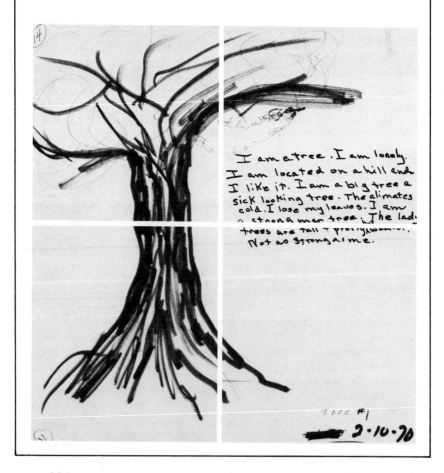

scribed her as "withdrawn and isolated; chronically depressed and indifferent to people and events."

During their first meeting, Lori told art psychotherapist Helen Landgarten: "I'm so happy to have a place to show all my problems and to be able to talk about them." However, when Lori was asked to draw what she was feeling, she said she could think of nothing. Finally, with a marking pen, she made a single halting black line on the paper. For the next few months, she was unable to describe specific problems; she spoke very little, often saying, "Nothing is happening."

When she finally began to draw, Lori's early pictures were filled with animals, fantasies of going somewhere, wishes for a peaceful society — and cash registers. The cash register, it appeared, represented Lori's major accomplishment: her cashier's job at school.

In the third month of treatment, Lori drew a tree and wrote: "I am a tree. I am lonely, I am located on a hill and I like it. I am a big tree, a sick looking tree. The climate is cold. I lose my leaves. I am a strong man tree. . . ." To the therapist, the picture and the description revealed Lori's identification with her father rather than with her nonfunctioning mother.

For a long time, Lori was unable to express anger. When Landgarten asked her to pick out six pictures of angry people and describe what they were thinking, Lori was vague and equivocal. It was not until the seventh month that Lori was able to identify in a nondirected collage a memory of anger at her sister — when Frances and her cousin had baked cookies and left none for her. "The remembrance of angry feelings was the first breakthrough of her denial system," writes Landgarten. "It was of particular importance due to the symbiosis which existed between Lori and Frances." Similarly, Lori had always described her mother as "nice." But a week after the "cookie" picture, Lori picked out a picture that she identified as her mother and described her as "grouchy and miserable," and "a lousy mother because she doesn't know how to discipline her own children and she acts childish."

With the support of the therapist, Lori made attempts at social involvements. She volunteered to do clerical work at the Red Cross, began guitar lessons at the YWCA, and she checked into several school clubs.

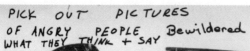

PICK OUT PICTURES
OF ANGRY PEOPLE   Bewildered
WHAT THEY THINK + SAY

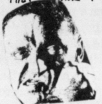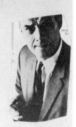

Would say: Blank
what I'd wish to say : what
are your feelings?

Would say : How's
your work doing
with you?
What I'd wish to
say :

He is a doctor

2/18/70

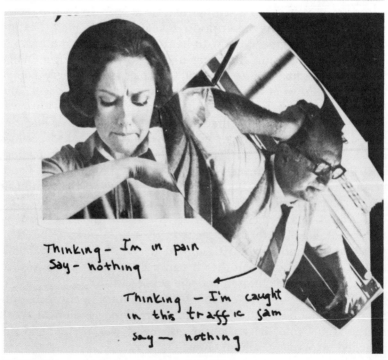

Thinking - I'm in pain
Say - nothing

Thinking - I'm caught
in this traffic jam
say - nothing

106

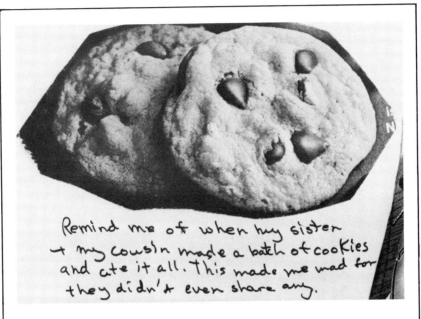

Remind me of when my sister + my cousin made a batch of cookies and ate it all. This made me mad for they didn't even share any.

About a year after treatment had begun, Frances left home, and Lori's pictures and descriptions became more revealing of her repressed feelings and her increased awareness. Following an incident in school in which the teacher complained about her and classmates spoke on her behalf, Lori drew a picture that she called: "People Always Talked for Me." She revealed that in school and even at home, Frances had spoken for her to the point where Lori had become, in effect, an elective mute. "She never spoke during the entire time she attended elementary and junior high school," Landgarten reported. "One teacher after another was informed that Lori did not speak. Therefore, neither the instructors nor students directed any communication to her."

At the end of sixteen months of treatment, Lori's pictures began to show positive elements. She drew "How I Feel Today," and wrote: "I feel happy, as if I have no real problems to be concerned over. People seem much more interesting than they ever have been to me before. I feel it's a great thing to be living." Within the next few months, Lori went on a diet and lost weight, and she began to use makeup and chose her own clothes. She was surprised and pleased by the compliments

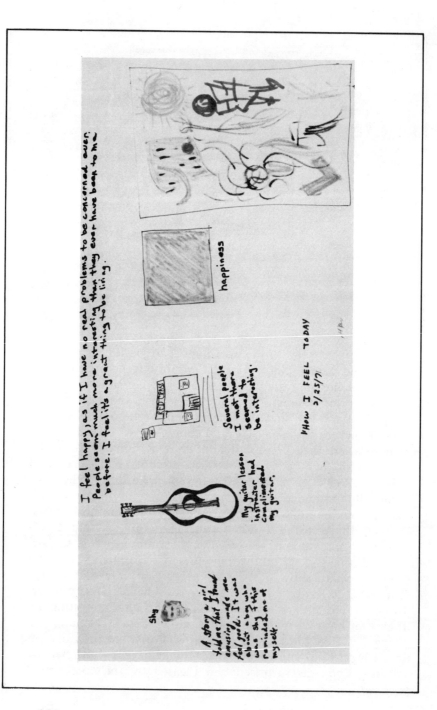

I feel happy, as if I have no real problems to be concerned over. People seem much more interesting than they ever have been to me before. I feel it's a great thing to be living.

happiness

Several people I met there seemed to be interesting.

My guitar lesson instructor had complimented my guitar.

Shy

A story a girl told me that I found amusing made me feel good. It was about a boy who was shy. The boy reminded me of myself.

►How I Feel Today 5/25/71

she received. In the twenty-fourth month of treatment, Lori found a part-time job in a dress shop and passed her driver's test.

About two years after treatment had begun, and just before Christmas, Lori was depressed: her mother had been hospitalized, and school was going badly. She drew a picture and then wrote about it: "Our house is dark; there is color everywhere else."

Helen Landgarten was going out of town during the holidays, and she gave Lori an assignment to continue painting and writing. The assignment would help maintain contact, and it would divert Lori's energies from depression to creativity. After the holidays, Lori reported:

> When I drew and then I started writing down what I felt, things began clearing up for me. I couldn't believe how much the art and writing every day helped me see how things really were. It began with Christmas — I painted several Christmas pictures. Those paintings really are merry and happy. I was so surprised at how very good Christmas turned out. As I thought and painted, I realized that it was because Frances wasn't there. In the past she would tell us all when to open the presents, when to eat and what to do. . . . Then there is this drawing with the eye in the middle and these wavy lines one after another making bigger and bigger circles. Suddenly I was like that eye observing. Seeing these people for the first time and how they acted, I was able to be in the room but be *separate from them!* . . .

During the last ten months of treatment, Lori began to date. Her pictures showed what she called "a state of confusion" and the need to "explore." At the end of January, Lori drew a self-portrait and wrote: "I see a change in myself. I see confidence and a willingness to stand up for myself and for others. I express my ideas more. . . . I told Frances how I felt about her!!! I also told a fellow I dated that he was rude. I stuck up for my dad when I thought he was right about something."

All of Lori's pictures had been in color. One day, however, she made a drawing in pencil that showed two figures lying in the sand. Lori admitted that she had had sexual relations with a date. Later, she said she had been concerned about the therapist's reaction, and, in a picture, she showed surprise at the

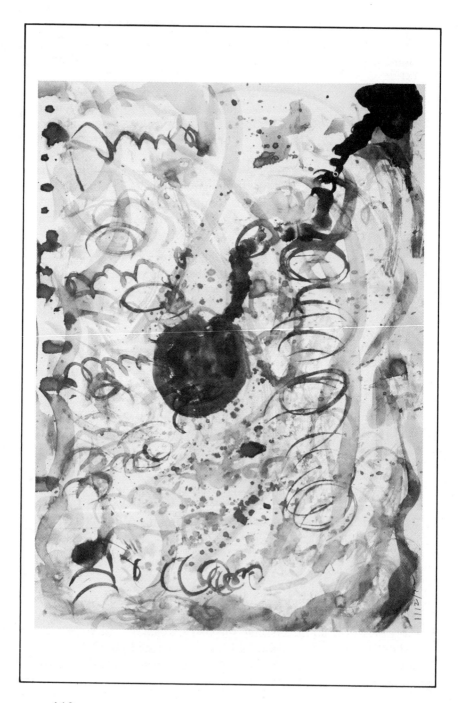

110

nonjudgmental response. In the next few weeks, Lori made new friends, began to associate "with people who I usually considered the least likely I would have associated with, namely marijuana smokers, drinkers, and bums (as they call themselves)." She felt a sense of satisfaction, but she also began to question her motives. "I'm beginning to wonder what I really do feel about John. I think I like him more than I thought I did or something. I feel wanted when I'm with him and his friends. *Maybe I'm using him as a substitute for the lack of love I have at home. I don't know.*" Lori's disappointment in her parents prompted a discussion in which Lori recognized that, in light of her mother's inability to cope with life on any level, it was unrealistic to expect meaningful interaction with her.

During the twenty-ninth month of art psychotherapy, Lori stopped dating her boyfriend, feeling that he was incapable of giving her a deep and close relationship. She saw his drug use as an escape and had come to think of him as a "loser."

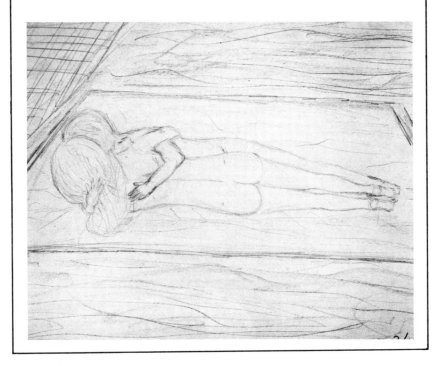

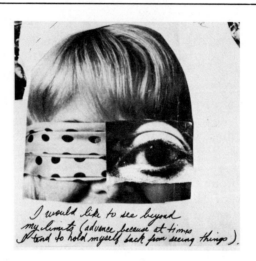

I would like to see beyond my limits (advance because at times I tend to hold myself back from seeing things).

In her last collage, after thirty-four months of art psychotherapy, Lori pasted a picture of a blindfolded girl and superimposed an open eye on one side of the blindfold. Underneath, she wrote a poem:

Looking Past the Shaded Bounds

There stands one child alone and blind. She has no lack of sight but yet she cannot see. Then in her life there appears a light. It is the inner glow which grows within her giving warmth, love, hope, desire — As she stands she begins to move at a pace slower than many. But she keeps pushing forth till she's pacing near, equal to those around.

The child has grown to near womanhood but she still has limits of sight — so pushing still she'll continue till she sees past these limits of sight.

Condensed from "Lori: Art Therapy and Self-Discovery," by Helen Landgarten, M.A., A.T.R., H.L.M.; Associate Professor and Director, Graduate Program in Clinical Art Therapy, Loyola Marymount University, Los Angeles, and Coordinator of Art Psychotherapy, Thalians Community Mental Health Center, Cedars-Sinai Medical Center. The complete case appears in Helen Landgarten, *Clinical Art Therapy* (New York: Brunner/Mazel, in press). The case is also the subject of a color and sound film produced by Professor Landgarten and is available from Art Therapy Film Distributors, 1141 Hartzell St., Los Angeles, CA 90272.

4

Music Therapy

Music occupies an ambiguous position in our Western culture. On the one hand, it represents pure emotion; on the other, the most refined elements of reason. Western attitudes toward music, as with so much in our culture, can be traced back at least as far as the Greeks, who put instruments in the hands of an incongruous pair of gods — Dionysus and Apollo.

Associated with Dionysus, or Bacchus, god of wine and orgies, was the concept of an unrestrained, wild, and undisciplined music that appealed to the senses. The mysteries associated with the Dionysian rites are marked by exhilaration, ecstasy, wild dancing, and throbbing music that arouses the senses and the emotions. These rites were said to have originated among the rude tribes of Thrace, "who were notoriously addicted to drunkenness."[1] But the surrender to pure emotion inherent in the Dionysian rites — the extravagant rituals, the near-savagery in the mysteries of Dionysus — found a willing audience throughout Greece. Reenacting the passion of Dionysus, his followers would tear a live bull to pieces with their teeth and roam the woods to the wild music of flutes and cymbals, engaging in orgiastic excesses.

In sharp contrast was the Greek music of logic, of perfect order, of harmony and balance. Pythagoras, the mathematician-philosopher, was intrigued with music as mathematics — a correlation that lasted until recent times. A tight string, he observed, would produce a "fundamental note" when plucked. But if that string were held in the center, each side would produce a note exactly an octave higher than the fundamental note; the two notes, though, would blend perfectly. If the string were held one-third of the way from either end, it would produce, on one side, a note a fifth higher than the fundamental note, and on the other side an octave and a fifth higher. All the way through the proportions, Pythagoras developed a mathematical projection of lengths and notes.[2] Pythagoras, in fact, made the bold claim that the universe itself was governed by mathematical principles, and he conjectured that the planets move in perfectly blended proportions and create, as they move, a "music of the spheres," or a "harmony of the universe."[3] It was appropriate that Apollo, the Greek god simultaneously of music and medicine, should have chosen Pythagoras, a practicing physician as well as a mathematician, to find in music this harmony that characterized order and well-being.

To the philosophers of the Middle Ages, it made sense that the music of the world, the *musica mundana*, was an instrument of God through which He provided for an earthly harmony and order. With the *musica humana*, the music through which the human soul was tuned to universal harmonies, the study of world music in the medieval universities was one of the seven liberal arts, a study of mathematical proportions and relationships. On the other hand, the medieval Church discouraged the instrumental music that was associated with the pagan rites, with the sensuousness of the dance, and with the profane stage. "It might be said," writes Joseph Kerman, "that Christianity converted the music of Apollo, god of light, reason and order, into the music of Christ. The music of Dionysus, god of wine and orgies, was very deeply buried — or consigned to hell, if we can believe the vivid painting by Jerome Bosch [in which the souls of the damned swirl around musical instruments]."[4]

In modern music therapy, we can discern both Dionysian and Apollonian elements. Music is a device for reaching into the emotions, for engaging the raw and sensitive edges of repressed feelings so that they can be drawn to the surface. More frequently, music is used to assuage, to soothe — but also to arouse and energize. In modern usage, the Apollonian concept prevails. Music is the restorer of equilibrium, of order and harmony with the world in which we live and with the people with whom we share it.

The use of music specifically for therapy is a relatively new phenomenon in this country. Before World War I, music was occasionally played to mental patients on the vague assumption that it activated the metabolic functions and stimulated the free working of the organs by relieving mental strain and emotional blockage. Between World War I and World War II, music was played largely as a general soporific and morale builder; it was a humane way for patients to while away their convalescence. The emphasis was on the healing and soothing powers of music, and the activity involved was listening. Accounts appeared in the popular press from time to time, reporting "miracle cures" that resulted from "reaching" patients through music when they responded to nothing else. There appeared to be a continuing belief that listening to music was itself therapeutic and that music had inherent healing properties.

THE RESEARCH BASE

The impetus for research in music therapy was the need to help the swelling populations of veterans' hospitals during and after World War II. The "talking cure," which had been the standard treatment for mentally disturbed patients, was no longer adequate or feasible in view of the large numbers of patients in hospital wards during the war. The energizing and tranquilizing drugs that were developed and used in mental health during the 1940s and 1950s were seen, at first, more as ways of making patients more amenable to psychotherapy than as treatments in themselves.[5] Similarly, music therapy was used, together with other "activity" programs, as "adjunctive" or "supportive" programs.[6] Challenged by hospital administrators, music therapists were forced to demonstrate the value of their work through empirical tests.

During the 1940s and 1950s, investigators began to probe the relationships between music, physiological changes, mood changes, and general mental health. It was found that listening to music produced changes in blood flow and blood pressure,[7] changes in posture,[8] pulse rate, and general activity of schizophrenics,[9] and breathing.[10] Researchers demonstrated that listening to music

produced measurable mood change[11] and that listening to and
playing music were effective antidepressant measures.[12]

Such studies persuaded the Veterans Administration to develop comprehensive music therapy programs at all VA hospitals —
a move which made the VA the acknowledged leader in the field
of music therapy. Since World War II, research in music therapy has
tended to center in the areas of specific problems, such as autism,
behavior disorders, mental retardation, and physical disorders. In
contrast with research in art therapy or dance/movement therapy,
research in music therapy tends to be more rigorously "scientific"
(probably one reason for the heavy behavioristic orientation in
music therapy) and to develop narrow bodies of findings in specific
areas on a pragmatic basis.[13] Little research seems to have had
wide theoretical applicability. However, given the concern for scientific validation, research in music therapy still leaves much to be
desired, according to some within the field. Donald E. Michel,
writing more than a decade ago, complained that "reports of experimental research [on the behavior disorders of children and
adolescents] are rare. A few articles illustrate objective observation
and evaluation of music therapy procedures, but others are pure
testimonials."[14] A survey of recent articles in the *Journal of Music
Therapy* reveals that contributions still consist of a mixture of experimental research findings, descriptions of programs, and hypotheses of treatments that *might* work. However, basic directions
in music therapy and underlying principles do emerge out of the
findings that have been reported.

In 1964, a group of eleven college and university teachers
of music therapy held a conference in Lawrence, Kansas, to evaluate
and consolidate the thinking and research in the field. The conferees
agreed to compile a basic collection of research and case studies
in music therapy, a project that was funded by a grant from the
U.S. Office of Education. That collection was subsequently expanded under the direction of E. Thayer Gaston of the University
of Kansas and published as *Music in Therapy* in 1968.[15] Despite
its age, it is still a basic reference in the field.

Considering the fact that fifty-nine individuals submitted
materials, it is remarkable that there was general agreement among
the contributors on the three basic principles to emerge from the
research. The consensus was that there are three ways in which music
can contribute to therapy:[16]

1. It can help individuals establish or reestablish interpersonal
   interactions and social involvements.

2. It can help individuals develop self-esteem through self-actualization.
3. The rhythmic structure of music can energize and bring order.

PSYCHOLOGICAL FOUNDATIONS
OF MUSIC THERAPY

The literature of music therapy seems to reveal a curious absence of direct and specific attempts to ground the theoretical framework of music therapy to psychological principles or psychotherapeutic theories — despite the fact that heavy borrowing can be inferred from the use of terms like "self-actualization" and "behavior changes through reinforcement."[17] There have been some few attempts, when music therapists were establishing their credentials for work in veterans hospitals, to relate music therapy to Freudian analysis. In 1945, for example, Isadore H. Coriat, writing in the *Psychoanalytic Review*, tried to persuade psychoanalysts that music's appeal to the individual had respectable roots in analytic principles. He stressed the repetition compulsion in music, contending that this compulsion appeals to the id's pleasure principle and overcomes the ego's governing reality principle, and he pointed to the symbolic content of music that could be interpreted analytically.[18] By and large, however, music therapy has been ignored by psychoanalysts, except as a sedative. Juliette Alvin, a leading British music therapist complains:

> The relationship between music and dreams, music and unconscious states has been observed throughout history. It is curious that the Freudian school has not paid more attention to this relationship. We all know how sound itself can affect our subconscious thoughts, and we are now seeing the development of techniques meant to use our conscious power of sound-retention during sleep.[19]

From the discussion of theory in the literature, it would appear that many music therapists have tended to view the field largely in terms of physiology; that is, in light of its influence on the body. However, the distinction between the physiological and the psychological is ambiguous. Art philosopher Susanne Langer contends that emotion is created by nervous excitement,[20] and music therapy pioneer Ira M. Altshuler attempts to trace the resocialization function of music to the way musical sounds reach and affect the nervous system.[21] Unlike researchers in dance/movement therapy, however, few music therapists appear to have explored this relationship between the physiological and the psychological in an attempt to develop a theoretical structure. Most of the research remains narrow, empirical, practical, and nontheoretical.

It seems reasonable to infer that the heavy physiological bias in music therapy and the absence of strong theoretical frameworks may be due in large part to the fact that music therapy in this country was developed largely by physicians in VA hospitals, and not — as was the case in the other expressive arts therapies — by practitioners in the arts. Consequently, music therapy adheres to the medical model perhaps more strongly than do the others. Moreover, the musicians brought in to do the actual work in the hospitals were generally music teachers, whose basic task was conceived to be the teaching of musical skills. The distinction between education and therapy in music appears to be more blurred than in any of the other expressive arts. The differences appear to exist less in what actually happens in the situation than in the fundamental goals of the practitioners. E. Thayer Gaston (who is a professor of music education, as well as the director of music therapy at the University of Kansas) writes:

> Perhaps music therapy and music education can best be distinguished by the fact that the music therapist is chiefly concerned with eliciting changes in behavior, not with perfecting musical endeavor. The opposite is true of the music educator. Characteristics of patients nearly always differ significantly from those of students. The music therapist is more sensitive to the *nonmusical* behavior of the child, the music educator to the *musical behavior* of the child. Even so, music therapy and music education have much in common.[22]

Nevertheless, there have been attempts to establish a clear theoretical base for music therapy. Two major directions emerge: (1) the development of a structure that is independent of psychological theory, and (2) the building of a framework that flows implicitly out of behaviorist psychology and behavior therapy. The two directions converge; much of the terminology, the technique, and the objectives in the "independent" theories seem to borrow heavily from behaviorism. The convergence is understandable since the independent approaches are generally viewed as educational, in the sense that they are aimed at changing the behavior of their clientele. Because behaviorists see their own work as reeducation more than as therapy, it is natural that the "independents" should have borrowed what they see as the more successful of the behaviorist techniques.

Describing the organization of research data and studies in his classic collection, Gaston writes: "Rather than explaining music therapy in terms of a particular psychological theory, we have made an effort throughout to show how music therapy can bring about desirable changes in behavior and adaptation."[23]

Gaston's reluctance to accept a behaviorist label is apparently based on his concern over the behaviorist rejection of "most of what makes life worth living, the 'feelingful' aspects." He believes that to set up constructs based *only* on observable behavior, constructs "that bear little relation to physiological function, for example, is to set up guidelines external to the organism."[24] Gaston pleads for a multidisciplinary approach, by which he means a combination of biodynamic, sociological, behavioral, and aesthetic research techniques and findings to support a discipline of music therapy. Aesthetics, which Gaston defines as a "science" rather than as a philosophy (quoting *Webster's Third New International Dictionary*), has much to offer music therapy. "Esthetic experience may be one of the best devices to help [man] adjust and adapt to his environment," Gaston says. "To understand 'humanness' is to understand more profoundly what is necessary for the health and happiness of man."[25] And music, he contends, is the essence of humanness, not only because it is created by man, but because man creates his relationship to it.

Gaston identifies rhythm as the most significant single element of music. It is an energizer as essential to music as the heartbeat is to human life; without rhythm, there could be no music. Rhythm is also an organizing instrument that serves to coordinate sound, to influence activity, to communicate, to structure reality, and — on a social level — to bring people together to dance, play, and listen. Rhythm serves to control behavior; it provides a nonverbal persuasion not only to act but to act in concert with others.[26] To rely exclusively on any psychology that ignores the aesthetic elements of music, therefore, would severely cripple music therapy.

However, despite Gaston's disavowal of dependence on a particular psychological theory, an examination of the specific programs described in his collection, and the research included, reveals that operationally, the majority are based squarely on behavioral models. Moreover, an examination of the lists of goals published by many hospitals and clinics for their music therapy programs reveals clearly behavioral goals expressed in behavioral terms. For example, one southern state hospital states in its literature that "music itself demands a definite structured behavior . . . that can be measured through time; at the same time it can be enjoyable (positively reinforcing), motivating, and relaxing."[27] Many of the institutional programs stress behavior changes that will accompany or result from regular voluntary attendance at the music sessions, obedience to the conductor's beat, or singing in time.[28]

The behaviorist influence seems to have been modified to a somewhat minor degree by practices and terminology that have leaked from humanism, as we shall see later in this chapter. In operation, music therapy seems to be more structured than any of the other arts therapies, and its methodologies approach those of music education. (See Tools of the Trade, p. 143.) Writes Donald Michel:

> Using the structuring aspect of music to organize learning, the reinforcing (reward) aspect to help change old behavioral patterns and shape new ones, or the social group aspect to develop interpersonal interaction and to structure appropriate involvement of individuals in social settings, the music therapist tends to work in much the same general way, whatever the problem or behavior disorder.[29]

MUSIC IN DIAGNOSIS

The value of a diagnosis rests on its validity — its ability to identify, measure, or predict what it purports to identify, measure, or predict. From observations of the patient's symptoms, the therapist infers the problem or the category of disorder, so that appropriate treatment can be prescribed.

Major problems persist in mental health diagnosis. One is that the categories — schizophrenia, neurosis, obsession — are very general constructs from which it is extremely difficult to predict how a given individual is likely to behave. The predictive validity of diagnosis in mental health is extremely low, as is evidenced by the common — and somewhat disconcerting — phenomenon of clashes of testimony among highly credentialed and well-trained therapists and psychiatrists on the potential danger involved in permitting a criminal to roam the streets. Measurement, in the sense of "how much" or "how serious" a disorder may be, is virtually nonexistent in mental health, given the absence of clearly defined and generally agreed-upon standards. So diagnosis in mental health usually means deciding on the appropriate label to use in categorizing the conglomerate of an individual's symptoms.

This last problem, in turn, is confused by the fact that the categories of disorder are extremely fuzzy around the edges. Therapists rarely deal with normality. Their patients come to them by virtue of their abnormalities, or deviations, or peculiarities. Unfortunately, few deviations lend themselves to neat categorization. For example, the concepts of schizophrenia, autism, and brain-damage are *disjunctive:* they are based on the personal judgments of the therapist as to whether the cluster of symptoms that the patient exhibits — or fails to exhibit — warrants a particular label.

This fuzziness has led many therapists to reject the notion of personal diagnosis altogether, on the ground that the application of labels may do more harm than good. Gestalt therapist Walter Kempler, for example, contends that labels "can astigmatize the vision of the next therapist who sees the chart before he sees the patient."[30] He believes that labels may be more useful in describing the therapist who has diagnosed than the patient who is being diagnosed. And William Glasser, the founder of reality therapy, argues that labels tend to distort because of varying definitions and understandings about what the labels mean.[31]

Nevertheless, most psychoanalytically oriented arts therapists, and most therapists of any persuasion who work in hospitals or clinics, continue to adhere to the nosology, or classification of disorders, that has evolved out of verbal clinical psychoanalysis. To correlate this admittedly imperfect system with a symptomology that arises in other contexts, as in music or art, adds additional dimensions of possible distortion. However, many music therapists contend that such independent assessments may also add dimensions of corroboration to diagnoses by psychotherapists or clinical psychologists. As a result, they have long sought some diagnostic clues that may arise in connection with their own work.

There have been two major areas of investigation in the attempt to use music diagnostically. The first and more common one is focused on the search for correlations. Do the music preferences of normal and disordered individuals differ? Do they perceive music differently? Are there music preference styles or patterns that are common to schizophrenics? To manics? To psychopaths?

During the 1950s, when music therapists were laboring to legitimize their work in VA hospitals, a number of investigators attempted to find just such correlations.[32] For a variety of reasons, the results were ambiguous. Even where positive correlations were found, they were not statistically "significant," for the most part.

Similar attempts in the United Kingdom were of limited usefulness. Two therapists, writing in the *British Monthly Review of Psychiatry and Neurology*, noted that patients' responses to music are often incongruous and unrelated to the nature of the music to which they listen. A neurotic, for example, would describe light, gay music as depressing or restless; a psychopath projected his own facade of defense — an unrelenting optimism — to the point where every piece was characterized as gleeful and joyful. The observers stated that "these incongruous responses often proved of some diagnostic value by throwing some light on the personalities of the patients, on their unconscious attitudes and conflicts, and thus indirectly were of value to psychotherapy."[33] However, no clear correlation was established between the type of response elicited and the specifics of the disorder.

For some years, researchers in the area of correlation have used the IPAT (Institute for Personality and Ability Testing) Music Preference Test, which consists of one hundred musical excerpts, in an attempt to provide the standard tasks that are necessary if patients and groups are to be compared with each other. Some investigators have been encouraged by results that have emerged. For example, in one study that involved a control normal group and six groups of patients who had been diagnosed as suffering a variety of emotional and organic disorders, not only was a difference found between the control group and the patient groups, but significant differences were found between the patient groups.[34] However, over the years, the overall results can best be described as equivocal and inconclusive.

The attempt to correlate diagnostic categories and music preference is not universally supported by music therapists. Donald E. Michel, for example, resists the whole notion of using category labels as diagnostic descriptions. Such labels, he asserts, are useful only for the convenience of those "who need a quick identification or grouping of persons with similar problems."[35] He contends that the therapist must look further than the label under which he finds a patient, because the labels may be misleading and because many patients, especially children, often suffer multiple handicaps. To Michel, the diagnosis of an individual's problem is best accomplished in the course of treatment, in which careful records are kept and changes that have taken place are measured and related to specific treatment.[36]

The other major thrust in the attempt to use music for diagnostic purposes has focused on the Freudian concept of projection, much as the Rorschach is used in art therapy and verbal therapy. Researchers have found that normal subjects and schizophrenics would tell markedly different stories after having listened to a range of musical excerpts,[37] that stories tended to be autobiographical and could reveal inner fantasies, illogical or disassociated thinking, and egocentricity,[38] and that interjudge reliability, or consistency, was high, both in terms of matching subjects and the stories they tell, and in connecting story types and diagnostic categories.[39]

Some investigators have attempted to establish the validity of musical-projection techniques by correlating patients' responses with the patients' scores on established personality tests, such as the *Minnesota Multiphasic Personality Inventory* (MMPI).[40] In light of the criticism of the MMPI itself and, indeed, of personality trait tests in general by most of the reviewers in the prestigious and respected *Mental Measurements Yearbooks*, such correlations seem questionable as a base for establishing validity.

In addition to the problems already mentioned, there are other serious limitations in using music for projective purposes. The projection itself is almost always verbal in nature, and the music is limited to stimulating the verbal response, much as the Rorschach elicits verbal responses — a limitation, as we have seen, that has persuaded many art therapists that the use of the Rorschach is not an art therapy technique, but a verbal one. But music projective devices lack even the qualities that may give the Rorschach some value in projection: its ambiguous, symmetrical, and neutral qualities. Music tends to provide external clues: it is happy or sad, fast or slow, melodic or dissonant.

The major drawback in the use of music in diagnosis, to many critics, is the fact that virtually all of the musical diagnostic techniques have been not only verbal, but indirect. Unlike the bulk of diagnostic techniques in art therapy or dance/movement therapy, the musical projective approaches elicit patient response rather than patient production. To many in the arts therapies and in the verbal therapies as well, this reliance on response robs diagnosis of its most valuable element: spontaneity or authenticity.

THE THERAPEUTIC
USE OF MUSIC

The general agreement on the function of music in therapy that Gaston's researchers explicated from their data has become the basic statement of function in music therapy. These three functions, therefore, will constitute the fundamental structure for our discussion of music in therapy.

Interpersonal Relationships

In the larger sense, that of establishing a relationship with the world outside of one's own skin, the socialization function of music seems to be the most important single function in music therapy. "Music is the most social of all arts," says Juliette Alvin. "It creates communication between people in infinite ways."[41] This theory seems to be true whether people are passively listening to music that is played to them or engaged in a group that is making music. Even at the most basic level — that of keeping silent when others are playing — the music experience imposes group standards. For those who play with others, the interaction is inescapable, more so than in any other art. In almost any gathering of people in which it is important to arouse a sense of community, of congeniality, or of spirit, we are likely to find music.

Music is nonthreatening interaction. Discussing self-conscious adolescents for whom verbal interaction may be difficult or even frightening, Wanda Lathom writes that even the cessation of talking when music is played offers relief from psychological stress. She says: "Because the musical activity can be structured to focus mainly on the activity rather than the interpersonal relationships, it can be a relatively nonthreatening means of working on more appropriate relationships."[42] It can also offer opportunities for a therapist to observe social interactions during situations in which the participants' self-consciousness is reduced.

For the patient, music may offer an escape from a closed world. Whatever its nature, Alvin points out, illness isolates the patient and at the same time threatens his or her identity, especially when the patient is hospitalized or depersonalized by the illness. A music group gives the patient an opportunity for self-assertion through the part for which he or she is responsible, and at the same time a sense of belonging to a group in which he or she is accepted. A music group — and most music therapy involves group activity — demands interpersonal cooperation, even when it begins with a one-to-one relationship. Alvin writes:

> There are many ways of using this one-to-one relationship technique leading to group relationship with musical means, even as simple as a single sound. We have recently watched a woman music therapist using primitive speaking African drums with a group of schizophrenic patients unable to communicate together. The varied pitch of these drums and their different

tone colour are striking; they seem to express different voices or personalities. The therapist began with a one-to-one relationship, one patient echoing on his drum the sound she had made on hers. At that stage other patients were drawn in one after the other. Each with his own drum and his own personal sound became part of the whole without losing his identity.[43]

In all the broad realm of disorders known as "behavior disorders"—those without an obvious physiologic basis—the use of music to draw the individual out of himself or herself is seen most dramatically in the case of autistic children and schizophrenics. Autism and some forms of schizophrenic disorder are characterized by a turning inward, a building of an unreal world around the individual, and the rejection of the real world that most of us know. This closed world may be a refuge, as Alvin points out, or it may be a prison. From this closed world come signals that we cannot understand—ritualistic, symbolic movements or postures that are bizarre to us.

Alvin contends that music may be the key to open the door—not so much for us to get inside the closed world, as to bring the patient out. "The depths where music can reach this patient," she writes, "are full of rituals, dreams and symbols, of obsessions, phobias and fantasies which are dissociated from the real perceptual world." Music can be the medium for the expression of these obsessions and phobias, so that they can become conscious and purposeful. "Then music can act as a means of communication, bringing the real and the unreal world together."[44]

The idea that music may be a key to the world of the autistic child is supported by findings that many such children are alert to musical elements. Autistic children have been reported to display unusual musical interest and ability, rote memory for melodies, and a preference for singing over speaking. Bernard Rimland, in his book, *Infantile Autism*, goes so far as to say that musical interest and ability are almost universal in autistic children.[45] In fact, some researchers suggest that there may be a direct connection between the autistic condition and this musical interest. One case is reported of an autistic child who, at eighteen months, could sing or hum songs by Schubert and Brahms as well as the themes of symphonies; as the child's condition improved, "his musical interest and ability waned, his accuracy diminished, and he sang less."[46]

Some are skeptical about the reports of a correlation between autism and musical interest or ability. Paul Nordoff and Clyde Robbins, of the University of Pennsylvania's Department of Psychiatry, suggest that the unusual preoccupation with music reported for autistic children may stand out because of the dearth of other interests, or because of the nonthreatening and nonpersonal nature of the experience. Referring to their own music therapy pilot project with twenty-six children, they report that there were a few indications of "freak musicality" in three children, but that "these proved to have no significance for treatment,"[47] Moreover, they report, because of the impaired communication system, it may be difficult to find the appropriate point of contact with music for a specific autistic child; many sessions may be spent just watching for a sign of recognition or interest, or for an indication of willingness to participate in music making.

However, they report some successes in their own work, and they describe some of the methodologies that seem to work. In one case report, music was used first to match or "mirror" the autistic child's own rhythm and then used as a lure to help her vary rhythm and tempo — an indication that she was aware of and responsive to outside stimuli.[48] This technique is strikingly similar to the "mirroring" of the movements of autistic children by movement therapists. In an expanded description of "matching," Nordoff and Robbins describe how a music therapist incorporates inadvertent or accidental sounds into a music structure and then feeds it back to the child in an effort to get him to respond and therefore establish a communication "circuit."[49]

Mary M. Wood, director of training of the Rutland Center in Georgia, tells of a group rhythm session in which a severely withdrawn schizophrenic boy tapped listlessly and randomly at his drum. Each time he made a sound, the therapist responded with a strong single beat from her drum. After several such responses, the boy looked up with a surprised expression, then broke into a wide grin. The two began to exchange beats. Reacting to the scene, Wood writes: "In a most vivid breakthrough this boy had recognized that the reciprocal beat was coming from her, in *response* to *him!* A first step in the process of social interaction had begun."[50]

Music therapists have found that the socialization function of music listening and music making is applicable to most types of patients. Working in groups necessitates the subordination of an individual's interests to those of the group. Moreover, the demand is impersonal, in the sense that it is imposed by musical considerations, not by another individual. Participation in a musical group provides a form of feedback for the individual on his or her own identity and accomplishments. It promotes a sense of being needed in the group as well as a sense of (and a scale for comparing) accomplishment and contribution. Most important, according to William Sears, it may spur the individual to further accomplishments if the experience is a positive one.[51]

Some research has been conducted in the kinds of experiences that encourage socialization. Even in simple music listening, it has been found that some kinds of music are more effective than others in promoting interpersonal relations. For example, romantic music does not seem particularly appropriate for this purpose; it tends to arouse personal associations and to create tensions. Far more effective in bringing people together and integrating a group are traditional and folk music selections.[52] A number of therapists are impressed with the improvement in group identity of hospitalized patients who participate in drum and bugle corps.[53]

While we began this section with the assertion that the socialization function may be the most important single function of music therapy, this statement is based more on an intuitive assumption by music therapists than on research data; remarkably little has been done on interfunction measurement or evaluation. Some studies and projects do tend to support this conclusion, though. For example, Daniel M. Weiss and Reuben J. Margolin, contrasting "music group therapy" (conducted as a music appreciation course) with verbal group therapy, found that the music experiences accent the resocialization function rather than the therapeutic one. The latter, they report, was better accomplished by analysis of personal problems.[54] Because of the somewhat narrow interpretation of music experiences in such studies, and because most reports on the socialization function have been presented as case histories or program descriptions rather than as findings derived from rigorously controlled experiments, a good deal of research must still be done in this area.

Self-Development
Anyone who thinks that the widespread use of terms like "self-development" and "self-actualization" by music therapists suggests a strong humanistic influence on music therapy is doomed to disappointment. The terms themselves have been transposed from the humanist movement and then have been redefined. As they are used in the literature of music therapy, they seem more comfortable in behaviorist than in humanist contexts. The terms are likely to mean the acquisition of skills in order to adapt to society. Describing self-development and self-actualization, Gaston writes:

There will have to be self-development . . . but always the eventual success will be in terms of the group. In each instance, it is the circumstance of environment that persuades the individual to change poor or inappropriate behavior for better behavior. And *behavior* used in this sense means anything that an organism does that involves action and response to internal or external stimulation. *This process of inducing behavioral changes is precisely what the music therapist brings about. . . . The therapist helps the patient to a healthier adaptation to society. . . .* The process of . . . [expanding horizons and widening perceptions] is self-actualization in greater degree and more meaningful participation in more significant groups. Thus one's life becomes broad and rich. Man does more than just cope with his environment — he lives expressively in his self and in his groups.[55]

To Gaston, self-development is clearly a means to an end. "The chief aim of therapy," he asserts unequivocally, "is to enable the individual to function at his best in society."[56] This goal can best be attained by helping the patient to change old habits, to learn new skills, and to substitute appropriate behaviors for the old maladjustive behaviors. The most effective methodologies for change, given this somewhat divergent view of self-development, are those of behavior modification. And, indeed, schedules of reinforcement — mostly positive, it should be noted — guide the day-to-day operation of most such programs. For the most part, it is assumed that the learning of the skills themselves — the ability to make music, the ability to deal with others in the course of making music or listening to it, the concomitant enhancement of self-esteem that is assumed to accompany the attainment of skills — are the behavioral objectives, or the "target behaviors," of the music therapy program.

The positive reinforcements may range from words of praise to the growth of self-esteem that accompanies recognition by others, or they may involve material rewards, or tokens of such reward, in a sophisticated system of deferred gratification. Thus, Donald Michel, who talks of increasing self-esteem through learning new music skills, describes motivation for such learning, as well as a method for charting progress, in terms of a token economy:

> One answer in some of today's hospitals is the development of "token-economy units," where each patient's behavior is made contingent by the use of tokens given for desired behaviors. This may exist for all patients at a rudimentary level of being "charged" tokens for beds and other basic comforts of living. Each patient has an individual chart which carries a record of all his behaviors and of his progress, largely in terms of tokens earned (or lost, i.e., "fined"). Music therapy's contribution more easily may be determined in terms of behaviors of the patient which are influenced through tokens charged or paid for.[57]

In recent years, a good deal of attention has been devoted to music *itself* as a reinforcement for desirable behavior. Both "contingent music" (playing music as a "reward") and "contingent interruption" of music (when behavior is "maladjustive") have been the focus of many studies. A group of experimenters used contingent music to reduce "inappropriate" behavior on school buses;[58] another used interrupted music to reduce the noise level in home economic classes;[59] and still another experimenter was able to subdue disruptive group behavior of emotionally disturbed boys.[60] One report claimed a significant reduction in the rate of multiple tics by resorting to "tic-contingent" interruption of music.[61] Several investigators report having used contingent music to improve mathematics skills[62] and to increase reading participation.[63]

The differences in the ways humanists use such terms as self-actualization and the ways in which the transplanted terms are used in music therapy become increasingly evident when we scratch the surface to identify the component elements of the concepts. According to Abraham Maslow, a major characteristic of the self-actualized person is his spontaneity.[64] And while spontaneous production receives considerable attention in the literature of art therapy and dance/movement therapy, it is rarely mentioned in music therapy.

There are probably several reasons for this neglect of spontaneity. For one thing, spontaneous or "authentic" production is valued by those who are psychoanalytically inclined as a form of self-revelation, an expression of unconscious feelings. But behaviorists, whose concern is overt, observable, and measurable behavior, have little regard for unconscious expressions; indeed, behaviorist theory has always been skeptical about the existence of an unconscious. Secondly, it is generally assumed that before someone can produce music at all, he or she needs to acquire musical knowledge and develop musical skills, a structured approach that inhibits spontaneous expression of anything but learned skills and practiced substance.

However, with new musical techniques, such as electronic music production, and with the acceptance of dissonant or even atonal music in the modern music world, there has developed a new therapy technique that makes it possible to bring music therapy somewhat closer in line with the spontaneous techniques of art and dance therapy. Juliette Alvin is intrigued with "the method of free atonal rhythmical improvisation by the individual or by a group, a technique sometimes called 'instant music' or 'collective improvisation,' according to the circumstances and for which no specific musical ability is needed when used as therapy."[65] In such therapy, each patient chooses his or her own instrument and — with neither conductor nor score — plays at whim. Describing such collective improvisation, Alvin writes:

> The free use of a musical instrument well directed is an excellent means
> for the patient who lives in an unreal world and cannot communicate.
> We should always bear in mind that for most of [these patients] vibrations
> of a musical sound act as a safe means of protection and projection. Many
> autistic or psychotic individuals use music in a timeless, trance-like way, as
> a means of escape in which reality, time or rules of behaviour do not exist
> or have disappeared.[66]

The spontaneity of such playing, writes Alvin, is virtually guaranteed by the fact that any ability a psychotic may have displayed previously often disintegrates with his personality. Consequently, "free improvisation may be a new musical experience not related to any failure or memory of the past, in which he can succeed in expressing himself."[67]

While such spontaneous production is expressive, it does not seem to suggest contact with the unconscious, as it would in visual art or dance; behaviorism and psychoanalysis are different games, played under different rules. From time to time, though, British music therapists write of spontaneous music making in ways that suggest a greater willingness than is apparent among their American counterparts to interpret in nonbehaviorist terms. Julienne Brown, describing music making by patients with no musical instruction or technique, writes in the *British Journal of Music Therapy:*

> Improvisation such as this is more than a musical experience. It puts us in
> direct touch with the dynamics of our emotional and intellectual inner
> lives. And this revelation is sometimes frightening and shocking, sometimes
> beautiful and rewarding.[68]

A somewhat divergent view of self-development in music therapy has developed in recent years that borrows more from child development and learning theories than from psychotherapeutic theories. Developmental music therapy, developed for use in special education, is described as a "psychoeducational" model that has brought together (1) assumptions from Piaget's theories of child development, (2) taxonomies, or classifications of educational objectives, (3) the expression of such objectives in behavioral terms, and (4) special education methodologies.[69]

Designed for use with emotionally disturbed children in learning situations, developmental music therapy identifies four curriculum areas (behavior, communication, socialization, and academics) and four stages of development (responding to music with pleasure, responding to music with success, learning music skills for successful group participation, and investing in group music processes). Richard M. Graham identifies a fifth stage: applying individual and group music skills in new situations.[70] Children are grouped by their developmental stage in each area, rather than by chronological age, and the approach rests on the principle of building on children's strengths, because it is assumed that even disturbed children can function normally in certain contexts and at certain times.

In operation, developmental music therapy seems to be more an educational than a therapeutic practice. However, like much of music therapy (and music education as well), it is heavily behaviorist in approach.

Energy and Order

Researchers in music therapy are fond of noting the almost irresistible demands that music makes on the body. Physical responses to music are obvious: we may find ourselves beating time to music; our breathing may speed up or slow down in time with passages to which we listen. The body responds to music in ways of which we may not even be aware. Investigators have measured the galvanic effects of musical vibrations on the skin,[71] changes in heart rate inspired by music,[72] and myriad other effects on the autonomic, or involuntary, system. It is commonly noted that the musical time unit in almost all cultures appears to be a standard that is roughly equal to the human heartbeat, between seventy and eighty beats a minute.[73]

The compelling interrelationship between the structured energy demands of music and the natural rhythms and responses of the body makes music a logical ordering instrument for certain kinds of problems, especially those in which coordination needs improvement. Gaston thinks that the energizing and ordering function is the most important one in music therapy for the mentally retarded and the physically handicapped.[74]

For some years, these rather obvious relationships between musical structure and natural rhythm have suggested therapeutic programs that are based on rather simple analogies. For example, if rhythm is ordered and uniform, then disturbed individuals who need order in their lives should listen to and make music so that they can become more structured. Until recent years, it has not been possible to verify that there has actually been any direct connection between musical order and that of the body. But within the past few decades, this situation has changed. The instruments now exist not only for verifying but for measuring the effects of music on the body and its functions: galvanic reaction, blood pressure, body movement, metabolism, and even electroencephalographic ("brain wave") patterns. As a result, a good number of studies have been directed toward demonstrating what had previously only been assumed: that music can influence the body in ways that are obvious and in ways that are not readily apparent.

Such findings, obviously, are useful in shaping hypotheses about how music might be used in therapy programs and in supporting the development of music therapy programs for the retarded and the physically handicapped. Many hypotheses have been advanced, and many programs have been developed — some, perhaps, in ways that are not readily supported by the research evidence to date.

The use of music with the mentally retarded has grown more quickly than any other therapeutic use of music, both in music therapy and in special education. In addition to the value of music in promoting socialization and in helping develop self-esteem, it is generally assumed that rhythm can help retardates develop a sense of structure and organization in their confused and chaotic private worlds. In fact, Betty Isern Howery contends that the order and structure of music provide the security that the retarded child needs for meaningful therapy. She writes that "the continuous basic beat and the repetition of the melodic structure provide an expectancy that will help alleviate the retardate's fear of the unknown."[75]

The therapeutic value of rhythmic music rests on the presumed transfer of the organizing and coordinating qualities of music to other areas of the individual's experience. Rhythmic work with such children, according to Valle Weigl, "facilitates coordination with others through the organizing, stimulative force of rhythm . . . [and] teaches them organization through the structure and genuine discipline inherent in musical form and rhythm."[76]

Based on a combination of transfer and repetitive experience, a number of programs have been organized to help retarded children improve their speech. Howery believes that music is highly effective in helping retardates master the developmental stages in the learning of speech in a nonthreatening and pleasurable way. She cites case data to support the contentions that vocabulary can effectively be expanded through the singing of songs and that memorization of data is more effective in connection with singing than with story-telling or rote.[77]

Music has been reported useful in helping retarded children coordinate muscular activity. It has even been credited with helping retarded children learn to write, first by capturing their attention, then by stimulating them to move rhythmically and freely, and finally by permitting them to progress to refined small motor movements, such as finger manipulation.[78]

The ordering quality of music has been the basis for a considerable amount of music therapy with physically handicapped children and adults, particularly those suffering from cerebral palsy, the disorder from which the largest single group of physically handicapped children in this country suffer. As with the mentally retarded, it has been reported that music is helpful in accelerating developmental progress. Therapists have claimed that music helps handicapped children learn sounds,[79] gain breath control,[80] and practice sound production by learning jingles and easy songs.[81]

On the basis of her own experiences with children suffering from cerebral palsy, Juliette Alvin cites both the energizing and the ordering effects of music. "I have noticed," she writes, "that music expressing movement can deeply reach a child who is chair-bound or lying on his back, not only from his immediate response but from a transfer of this emotion into another means of expression," as in drawings that show a good deal of movement.[82] Not only can the music itself help the child regulate and coordinate his music, but the playing of various instruments can help in the coordination of specific groups of muscles and responses.[83]

Several writers point out that the ordered quality of the music itself can be enhanced by providing a setting for music making that is itself highly structured. Wanda B. Lathom, director of music therapy at Parsons State Hospital in Kansas, writes:

> Within our society, marching and playing a field drum or a bass drum usually are perceived as masculine activities. They are, therefore, appealing to some adolescent boys who are trying to express their masculine identification. Because a drum corps marches in step and formation and plays a repetitive cadence, the structure is established to the fraction of a second. As it marches on the hospital grounds, other people stop to watch, and soon the members may have pride in their ability as a group. At this point, there may be considerable peer pressure for members to conform in order to give the group a uniform appearance.[84]

Reports testify to similar applications of the ordering quality of music with patients suffering from sight, hearing, speech, and other impediments. But the compelling rhythmic qualities of music can be disruptive as well as ordering. Beatrice Fields, working with brain-damaged adults, found that unless the rhythms are carefully matched with the patient's "capacities for neuromuscular activities," the resultant disharmonies can create tensions, anxieties, and even fears.[85]

Unfortunately, the bulk of the evidence on the success of music therapy in helping patients achieve order and structure in their activities is anecdotal in nature. It is described in the form of case histories or descriptions of music therapy programs. Virtually all of the experimental research in this area has been concentrated in the descriptions of the relationship between music and body rhythms: heartbeat, blood pressure, and so on. Very little controlled experimental research has been *evaluative* — that is, the determination of whether a program actually accomplishes what it is designed to accomplish and how well it does so compared with other forms of therapy, or no therapy at all. Until research in the area of outcome studies catches up with the proliferation of programs, such programs will be built largely on untested assumptions, anecdotal evidence, and hope.

Sedation

As in the case of art therapy, we propose the function of sedation with some hesitancy, largely because there are many who question whether sedation is, in fact, therapy. Nevertheless, it is mentioned so frequently in the literature of music therapy, and is the subject of so much research, that it demands some attention.

You may recall that one of the earliest applications of music therapy was sedation. David played his harp so that "the evil spirit" would depart from Saul, and Ambroise Paré calmed his more disturbed patients by having them listen to music. The first major use of music in this country for therapeutic purposes was designed to sedate and relieve.

With the scientific emphasis that began to pervade the music therapy field during and after World War II, a number of studies were designed to validate the sedative effects of music. In 1941, for example, Ira M. Altschuler and Bessey H. Shebesta compared the use of music alone and in conjunction with hydrotherapy for quieting disturbed patients. They found that music was as effective as hydrotherapy in tranquilizing disturbed schizophrenics. But because music can be played to large groups, they suggested that it may be more practical than hydrotherapy in sedation.[86] And Dr. Werner Simon demonstrated that the effects of music therapy programs — including both listening to and playing music — were almost as dramatic as those obtained by the administration of amphetamines for depression.[87]

In the 1950s, several researchers found that playing music in operating rooms before and during surgery allows the reduction of heavy sedation,[88] helps to reduce fear and anxiety in the patient prior to surgery, and helps alleviate tension in operating-room personnel.[89] One study underlined what might have appeared to be obvious, by concluding that sedative orchestral music was the most calming and that martial music and hymns were the least effective — probably for quite different reasons.[90]

Relatively little research has been reported in this area in very recent years, possibly because listening to music — especially piped-in music, as in an operating room or a recovery room — hardly demands the expertise of a trained music therapist.

CURRENT ISSUES IN
MUSIC THERAPY

Almost from the beginning of its modern development, music therapy marched off in a different direction than did art therapy and dance/movement therapy. Unlike the case in the other arts therapies, it was introduced into hospitals by physicians, rather than by artists. When musicians were brought into these hospitals, they came as performers or — more frequently — music teachers, rather than as therapists; music therapists had to fight for recognition in the arena of medical practice. As a result, they tended to justify their discipline by adhering to a rigorously "scientific" approach, usually correlated with behaviorism.

Developments in medicine, however, have converged with trends in the humanistic psychotherapies in some interesting respects. Humanists, who reject the medical model in therapy, have long sought to establish a community base for therapy to replace the traditional hospital program. Currently, the trend in mental health care facilities has been toward the establishment of community centers, most of them outpatient. They may be called, variously, halfway houses, community mental health centers, or day treatment centers. In addition, the growth of private nursing homes and residential centers for the aged, the handicapped, and the disturbed has been dramatic. In part, this trend has been the result of economic pressures; with the rocketing costs of hospitalization, the expense of maintaining patients in large state hospitals has simply been more than legislatures are willing to bear.

Many patients who are not considered dangerous to themselves or to society have been returned to their communities for any intermediate treatment that the community may be willing to provide. However, the trend is not merely a cold-hearted economic expediency. Rather, it reflects a growing recognition that the hospitalization of patients may actually aggravate their problems and hinder their recovery. Charles E. Braswell, applauding the development of the community facility, points out that "there is more than a chance relationship between social isolation and behavioral disorders."[91] Underlying the trend, he sees a basic shift from the traditional medical *reconstructive* approach to a *supportive* social adaptation model.

Among the advantages claimed for community-based programs are the following contentions:[92]

1. They provide structured programs outside the institution, thereby keeping intact the family and community ties of the patient.
2. The patient and the family avoid the shame associated with institutionalization, and a further diminution of self-esteem.
3. Day treatment status implies trust in the patient's ability to function in a society.
4. Day treatment provides the opportunity for a gradual reintegration into the community.

The trend toward community-based, mental health care, together with current trends toward shorter stays in mental hospitals (except for those considered severely regressed or dangerous to themselves or to others), and the phenomenal growth of nursing homes and residential centers, suggest that music therapists must be flexible in dealing with new support roles and short-term, community-related goals. Describing her work in the Milwaukee County Mental Health Center's day hospital program for retarded adults, Bonnie Wolfgram notes the high incidence of psychosis among her patients. She lists the major objectives of her music therapy program as the alleviation of psychotic symptoms, education and reinforcement of self-care and grooming skills, the development of behavioral controls, and the restoration of self-esteem. Underlying the program was the single major long-range goal: the reduction of the dependency of the patients, so that they can be integrated into the community.[93]

By and large, the community mental health approach is based on a modified medical model. However, some music therapists have moved further toward the broad educational model of the humanists. For example, Michel sees the ideal situation as one in which parents could bring children to learn how to continue in the home the therapy provided by expert therapists in the clinic. While this ideal situation is seldom encountered, he notes with approval the development of community-settlement-type schools in which music therapy is often provided. In community-based programs, he sees a trend toward the serving of persons with "ordinary" as well as those with "special" needs, thus providing a bridge for interaction between age groups and varied socioeconomic, racial, and ethnic groups in a community.[94]

Michel writes that "the future of music therapy definitely lies in the mainstream of the health-related services rather than in traditional institutions."[95] He sees future music therapists working in special education programs, in rehabilitation centers for the physically handicapped, and in programs for the disadvantaged. The music therapist, he asserts, can no longer be regarded merely as a *therapist*, but as a teacher as well.[96]

The convergence of the goals and methods of music therapy and music education is seen most clearly in the growth of Developmental Music Therapy. While this approach focuses on the needs of exceptional children, it does so by dealing with those elements of these children that are "normal"—suggesting a confluence, not only of therapy and education, but of humanist goals and behaviorist methods. The approach in music therapy is likely to be more eclectic than it has been in the past.

REFERENCE NOTES

1. James G. Frazer, *The New Golden Bough*, ed. Theodor H. Gaster (New York: Criterion Books, 1959), p. 351.
2. H. W. Janson and Joseph Kerman, *A History of Art and Music* (Englewood Cliffs, N.J.: Prentice-Hall, n.d.), p. 215.
3. Ibid.
4. Ibid., p. 217.
5. Stanley Boucher, unpublished lecture quoted in Donald E. Michel, *Music Therapy* (Springfield, Ill.: Charles C Thomas, 1976), p. 10.
6. Michel, *Music Therapy*, p. 8.

7. Margaret S. Sears, "A Study of the Vascular Changes in the Capillaries as Effected by Music" (master's thesis, University of Kansas, 1954).
8. William W. Sears, "Postural Response to Recorded Music" (master's thesis, University of Kansas, 1951).
9. Leo Shatin, "The Influence of Rhythmic Drumbeat Stimuli Upon the Pulse Rate and General Activity of Long-Term Schizophrenics," *Journal of Mental Science* 103 (January 1957):172-88; Clyde G. Skelly and George M. Haslerud, "Music and the General Activity of Apathetic Schizophrenics," *Journal of Abnormal and Social Psychology* 47 (April 1952):188-92.
10. Douglas S. Ellis and Gilbert Brighouse, "Effects of Music on Respiration and Heart-Rate," *American Journal of Psychology* 65 (January 1952): 39-47.
11. E. Thayer Gaston, "Dynamic Music Factors in Mood Change," *Music Educators Journal* 37 (February 1951):42-44; Robert Franklin Burns, *A Study of the Influence of Familiar Hymns on Moods and Associations: Potential Application in Music Therapy* (master's thesis, Florida State University, 1958).
12. Félix Marti-Ibañez, "Psychic Muse: Music, the Dance, and Medicine," *MD* 20 (October 1976):14-15.
13. E. Thayer Gaston, Erwin H. Schneider, and Robert F. Unkefer, *Music in Therapy*, ed. E. Thayer Gaston (New York: Macmillan, 1968), pp. 2-3.
14. Donald E. Michel, "The Psychiatric Approach and Music Therapy," in Gaston, *Music in Therapy*, p. 177.
15. Gaston, *Music in Therapy*.
16. Ibid., p. 4.
17. Michel, *Music Therapy*, p. 70.
18. Isadore H. Coriat, "Some Aspects of a Psychoanalytic Interpretation of Music," *Psychoanalytic Review* 32 (October 1945):408-18.
19. Juliette Alvin, *Music Therapy* (New York: Basic Books, 1975), p. 151.
20. Susanne Langer, *Philosophy in a New Key* (Cambridge, Mass.: Harvard University Press, 1963), p. 227.
21. Ira M. Altschuler, "The Part of Music in Resocialization of Mental Patients," *Occupational Therapy and Rehabilitation* 20 (April 1941):75-86.
22. Gaston, *Music in Therapy*, p. 292.
23. Ibid., p. 4.
24. Gaston, "Man and Music," in Gaston, *Music in Therapy*, pp. 7-9.
25. Ibid., p. 15.
26. Ibid., pp. 17-27.
27. Quoted in Michel, *Music Therapy*, p. 70.
28. Alvin, *Music Therapy*, p. 126.
29. Michel, *Music Therapy*, p. 51.
30. Walter Kempler, "Gestalt Therapy," in *Current Psychotherapies*, ed. Raymond Corsini (Itasca, Ill.: F. E. Peacock, 1973), p. 275.
31. William Glasser and Leonard M. Zunin, "Reality Therapy," in Corsini, *Current Psychotherapies*, p. 308.

32. Raymond B. Cattell and Jean C. Anderson, "The Measurement of Personality and Behavior Disorders by the IPAT Music Preference Test," *Journal of Applied Psychology* 37 (December 1953):446–54; Seymour Fisher and Rhoda Lee Fisher, "The Effects of Personal Insecurity on Reactions to Unfamiliar Music," *Journal of Social Psychology* 34 (November 1951): 265–73.
33. A. Zanker and M. M. Glatt, quoted in Alvin, *Music Therapy*, p. 139.
34. Raymond B. Cattell and R. E. McMichael, "Clinical Diagnosis by the IPAT Music Preference Test," *Journal of Consulting and Clinical Psychology* 24 (1960):333–41.
35. Michel, *Music Therapy*, p. 17.
36. Ibid., pp. 16–19.
37. L. Van Den Daele, "A Music Projective Technique," *Journal of Projective Techniques* 31 (1967):47–57.
38. Dorothy Brin Crocker, "Music as a Projective Technique," in *Music Therapy, 1955*, ed. E. Thayer Gaston (Lawrence, Kan.: The Allen Press, 1956).
39. Susan Grossman, "An Investigation of Crocker's Music Projective Techniques for Emotionally Disturbed Children," *Journal of Music Therapy* 15 (Winter 1978):179–84.
40. Andrew L. Sopchak, "Relation Between MMPI Scores and Musical Projective Test Scores," *Journal of Clinical Psychology* 13 (April 1957): 165–68.
41. Juliette Alvin, *Music for the Handicapped Child* (London: Oxford University Press, 1976), p. 53.
42. Wanda B. Lathom, "The Use of Music Therapy with Retarded Patients," in Gaston, *Music in Therapy*, p. 72.
43. Alvin, *Music Therapy*, p. 127.
44. Ibid., p. 138.
45. Bernard Rimland, *Infantile Autism* (New York: Basic Books, 1975), p. 127.
46. A. C. Sherwin, "Reactions to Music of Autistic (Schizophrenic) Children," *American Journal of Psychiatry* 109 (1953):823–31, quoted in Jo Ann Euper, "Early Infantile Autism," in Gaston, *Music in Therapy*, p. 186.
47. Paul Nordoff and Clyde Robbins, "Improvised Music as Therapy for Autistic Children," in Gaston, *Music in Therapy*, p. 192.
48. Ibid.
49. Paul Nordoff and Clyde Robbins, *Music Therapy for Handicapped Children* (New York: Steiner Publications, 1965).
50. Mary M. Wood, foreword to Jennie Purvis and Shelley Samet, *Music in Developmental Therapy: A Curriculum Guide* (Baltimore: University Park Press, 1975).
51. William W. Sears, "Processes in Music Therapy," in Gaston, *Music in Therapy*, p. 41.
52. Mitchell, quoted in Alvin, *Music Therapy*, p. 135.

53. Art Wrobel, "A Drum and Bugle Corps for Neuropsychiatric Hospital Patients," *Recreation* 48 (October 1955):392-93; Carol H. Bitcon, "The Drum Corps as a Treatment Medium," in Gaston, *Music in Therapy*, pp. 92-95.

54. Daniel M. Weiss and Reuben J. Margolin, "The Use of Music as an Adjunct to Group Therapy," *American Archives of Rehabilitation Therapy* 1 (March 1953):13-26.

55. Gaston, "Man and Music," p. 26.

56. Ibid., p. 27.

57. Michel, *Music Therapy*, p. 78.

58. Bonnie C. McCarty, Colleen T. McElfresh, Sheila V. Rice, and Susan J. Wilson, "The Effect of Contingent Background Music on Inappropriate Bus Behavior," *Journal of Music Therapy* 15 (Fall 1978):150-56.

59. C. W. Wilson and B. L. Hopkins, "The Effects of Contingent Music on the Intensity of Noise in Junior High Home Economics Classes," *Journal of Applied Behavior Analysis* 6 (1973):269-75.

60. S. B. Hauser, "Group Contingent Music Listening with Emotionally Disturbed Boys," *Journal of Music Therapy* 11 (Winter 1974):220-25.

61. B. H. Barrett, "Reduction in Rate of Multiple Tics by Free Operant Conditioning Methods," *Journal of Nervous and Mental Disease* 135 (1962): 187-95.

62. D. M. Miller, L. G. Dorow, and R. D. Greer, "The Contingent Use of Music and Art for Improving Arithmetic Scores," *Journal of Music Therapy* 11 (Summer 1974):57-64; C. K. Madsen, R. S. Moore, and J. U. Womble, "The Use of Music Subject Matter Versus Television as Reinforcement for Correct Mathematical Responses," *Journal of Research in Music Education* 24 (1976):51-59.

63. A. L. Steele and H. A. Jorgenson, "Music Therapy: An Effective Solution to Problems in Related Disciplines," *Journal of Music Therapy* 8 (Fall 1971):131-45.

64. Abraham Maslow, *Motivation and Personality* (New York: Harper & Row, 1954).

65. Alvin, *Music Therapy*, pp. 107-08.

66. Ibid.

67. Ibid., p. 108.

68. Quoted in Alvin, *Music Therapy*, p. 105.

69. Richard M. Graham, "Seven Million Plus Need Special Attention: Who Are They?" *Music Educators Journal* 58 (April 1972):24; Richard M. Graham, "Music Education of Emotionally Disturbed Children," in *Music for the Exceptional Child*, comp. R. M. Graham (Reston, Va.: Music Educators National Conference, 1975); Mary M. Wood, ed., *The Rutland Center Model for Treating Emotionally Disturbed Children*, 2nd ed. (Athens, Ga.: Technical Assistance Office, Rutland Center, 1972); Mary M. Wood, ed., *Developmental Therapy* (Baltimore: University Park Press, 1975); Jennie Purvis and Shelley Samet, *Music in Developmental Therapy: A Curriculum Guide* (Baltimore: University Park Press, 1975).

70. Graham, "Music Education of Emotionally Disturbed Children."
71. S. Podolsky, "Effects of Music on the Heart," in *Music Therapy*, ed. S. Podolsky (New York: Philosophical Library, 1954).
72. Ibid.; D. Ellis and G. Brighouse, "The Effects of Music on Respiratory and Heart Rate," in Podolsky, *Music Therapy*.
73. Alec Harman, *Man and His Music* (London: Barrie and Rockliff, 1962).
74. Gaston, *Music in Therapy*, p. vii.
75. Betty Isern Howery, "Overview," Part II: "Music Therapy for Mentally Retarded Children and Adults," in Gaston, *Music in Therapy*, p. 51.
76. Valle Weigl, "The Rhythmic Approach in Music Therapy," in *Music Therapy, 1962*, ed. Erwin H. Schneider (Lawrence, Kan.: The Allen Press, 1963), p. 80.
77. Betty Isern Howery, "Music Therapy for the Severely Retarded," in Gaston, *Music in Therapy*, pp. 58-60.
78. Louise W. Fraser, "The Use of Music in Teaching Writing to the Retarded Child," in *Music Therapy, 1960*, Erwin H. Schneider, ed. (Lawrence, Kan.: The Allen Press, 1961), pp. 66-89.
79. E. E. Doll, "Therapeutic Values of the Rhythmic Arts in the Education of Cerebral Palsied and Brain-Injured Children," in *Music Therapy, 1960*, pp. 79-85.
80. Valle Weigl, "Functional Music with Cerebral Palsied Children," in *Music Therapy, 1954*, ed. E. Thayer Gaston (Lawrence, Kan.: The Allen Press, 1955), pp. 135-43.
81. H. Westlake, "A System for Developing Speech with Cerebral Palsied Children," *Crippled Child* 29 (1951):9-11, 28-29.
82. Alvin, *Music for the Handicapped Child*, p. 114.
83. Ibid.
84. Lathom, "The Use of Music Therapy with Retarded Patients," p. 72.
85. Beatrice Fields, "Music as an Adjunct in the Treatment of Brain-Damaged Patients," *American Journal of Physical Medicine* 33 (October 1954): 273-83.
86. Ira M. Altschuler and Bessey H. Shebesta, "Music — An Aid in Management of the Psychotic Patient," *Journal of Nervous and Mental Disease* 94 (August 1941):179-83.
87. Marti-Ibañez, "Psychic Muse," p. 15.
88. G. A. Light, D. M. Love, D. Benson, and E. Trier Mörsch, "Music in Surgery," *Current Researches in Anesthesia and Analgesia* 33 (July/August 1954):258-64.
89. Kenneth L. Pickrell, James T. Metzger, N. John Wilde, T. Ray Broadbent, and Benjamin F. Edwards, "The Use and Therapeutic Value of Music in the Hospital and Operating Room," *Plastic and Reconstructive Surgery* 6 (August 1950):142-52.
90. Ibid.
91. Charles E. Braswell, "Social Facility and Mental Illness," in Gaston, *Music in Therapy*, p. 365.
92. M. I. Herz, "Day Hospitalization as an Alternative to Inpatient Hospital-

ization," in *Proceedings of the Annual Conference on Partial Hospitalization*, eds. R. Luber, J. Maxey, and P. Lefkowitz (Atlanta, Ga., 1976): pp. 105-06.

93. Bonnie J. Wolfgram, "Music Therapy for Retarded Adults with Psychotic Overlay: A Day Treatment Approach," *Journal of Music Therapy* 15 (Winter 1978):199-206.

94. Michel, *Music Therapy*, pp. 72-75.

95. Ibid., p. 117.

96. Ibid., pp. 115-16.

THE PREBAND INSTRUMENTS

Because the major purpose of music therapists is not usually to teach proficiency in music making or skill in playing the sophisticated band or orchestra instruments, they often turn to the same preband instruments that are used in early childhood education. These tools are the classroom instruments that click, and ring, and chime, and clang, and jingle. Such instruments are used for a wide variety of purposes: for instance, to develop sound discrimination and sharpen perception, to establish a sense of rhythm and order, and to promote social interaction in simple bands. Descriptions of some of the more common and frequently used preband instruments follow:

DRUMS

The percussive sound seems to satisfy a basic need, perhaps because of the awesome influence of the human heartbeat in our development. (The vast majority of mothers — both right-handed and left-handed — cradle their babies in their left arms, apparently because of the calming influence of the rhythmic heartbeat.) Drums of a variety of types — some beaten by hand, some struck with mallets or sticks — are basic tools of music therapy.

TAMBOURS AND TAMBOURINES

Tambours and tambourines are actually shallow hand drums. Tambourines have metal jingles anchored into slots that are cut into the wood shells. They may be struck by hand, or they may be shaken to produce just the jingling sound.

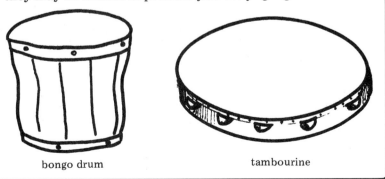

bongo drum   tambourine

WOOD-TONE INSTRUMENTS

Wood-tone instruments are usually held in the hand and struck, shaken, scraped, or rubbed.

Sand blocks are faced with abrasive materials that produce either "swishing" sounds when they are rubbed together or gourd sounds when they are struck together.

Claves and wood blocks (or tone blocks) produce sharp, clear clicks. Claves are hand-held rhythm sticks that are struck together, while wood blocks and tone blocks are struck with mallets.

Maracas are hollow gourds or wooden balls mounted on handles. They are partially filled with lead shot, dried seeds, or

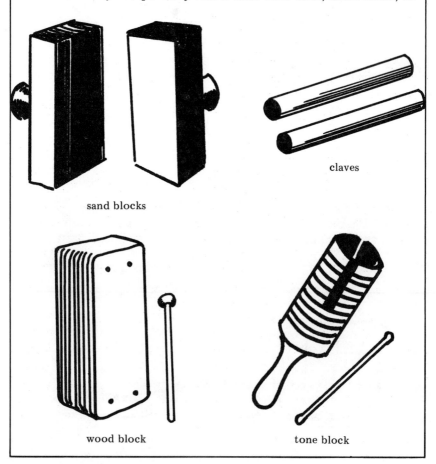

sand blocks

claves

wood block

tone block

small pebbles so that they can be used to produce a rhythmic beat when shaken.

Guiros are ribbed hollow instruments, carved either from cowhorns or from wood. They are scratched rhythmically with thin tapered sticks or with joined steel prongs to produce a rasping sound.

BELLS

Bells come in many forms — they may be metal bars, wooden bars, metal tubes, or perforated hollow balls. Some are shaken or swung, others are struck with hammers, fingered on a keyboard, or jingled when worn on wrist or ankle bands. Bells can be used either to alert and to energize or to relax.

Resonator bells are tone bars mounted on hollow wood resonator blocks. Struck with mallets, the resonator bells are separately tuned and may be played as a chromatic bell set by one person, or they may be distributed among the members of a group so that each player can strike one tone.

Song bars, or *melody bars*, are actually resonator bells that are mounted in sets of varying quantities and tones.

Jingle bells are simple pierced metal bells that contain metal pellets. They may be mounted on wrist straps, ankle straps, or on handles.

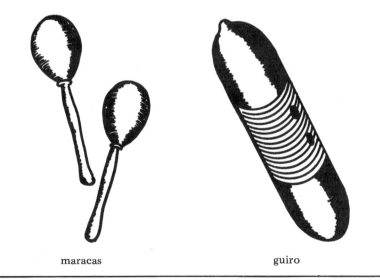

maracas   guiro

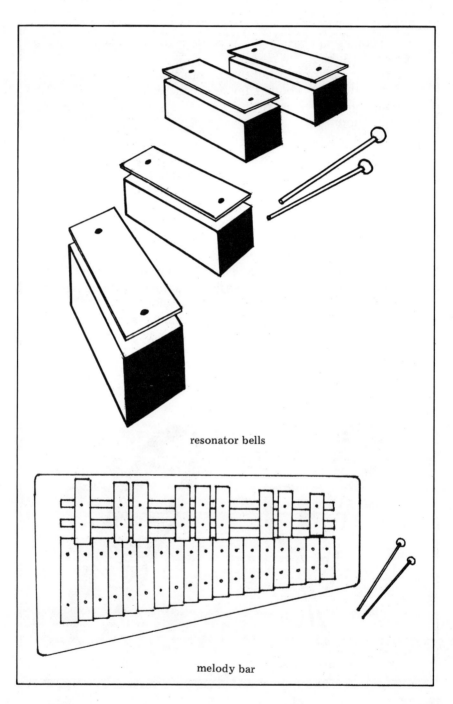

resonator bells

melody bar

146

A year later, after weekly therapy sessions, these photographs were taken during one session. The comments are those of Sister Mariam Pfeifer.

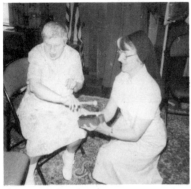 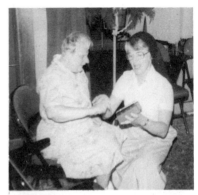

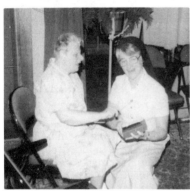 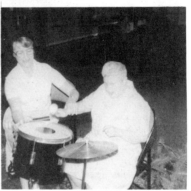

Following the song of greeting accompanied on the piano, E experiences the timbre of the resonator bells. She accepts the mallet from the therapist and begins to play in a chaotic manner.

As E increases her auditory perception, she improves her body alignment and faces the sound source. With minimal assistance, she plays the F and B^b resonator bells in a more acceptable fashion.

The pure sound of the bells prompts E to sing "Hello" as she plays. When she finishes, she returns the mallet to the music therapist with a pleasant "thank you." Previously, she had thrown the mallet or dropped it to the floor.

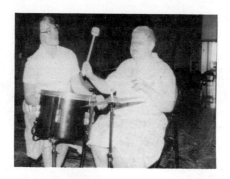

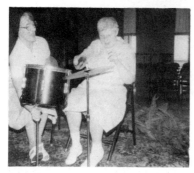

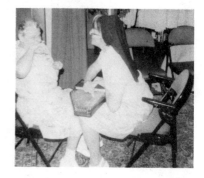

Sister Mariam Pfeifer uses the words "drum" and "cymbal" as she helps E find each instrument and strike it to identify the sound. This action is for the purpose of increasing vocabulary while developing auditory discrimination.

The drum activity gives E an opportunity to express her inner feelings and to vent her pent-up anxieties and tensions. This activity is an application of the third basic principle of music therapy, that of using rhythm to energize and bring order. E's attention span has increased considerably by this time. She has progressed from striking three or four erratic drumbeats and then throwing the mallet, to an involvement with the sound. She now plays as many as sixty-four measures, while she sings to the piano improvisation that is being played by a music therapy intern.

E crosses over from the drum to the cymbal to punctuate each verse with a crash. This engagement in sound, which brings about a crossing of the midline of the body, develops balance and space perception.

154

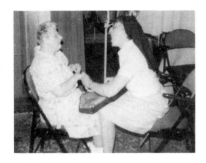 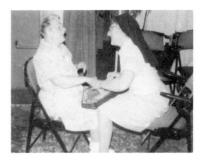

E still engages in momentary displays of self-abusive behaviors. Here, as the music activities change, E bites her hand. However, there has been a noticeable decrease in such inappropriate behaviors during music therapy sessions.

The music therapist quickly redirects E's activity from handbiting to holding a spatula, which is used here as a plectrum. E begins strumming the autoharp, with some assistance from the therapist.

E sings with the therapist, who has woven E's favorite phrases (once bellowed in a deep voice) into simple songs, in which they have been incorporated into meaningful sentences. E enjoys singing her pet phrases and has learned to use appropriate pitch; at the same time, the singing seems to have improved her general speech and communication skills. Music therapy seems to be the highlight of E's week, and other staff are impressed with E's progress in communication.

Adapted from an unpublished report prepared by Sister Mariam Pfeifer, I.H.M., M.A., R.M.T., music therapist, St. Joseph's Children's and Maternity Hospital, Scranton, Pennsylvania, and Northeast Tri-County Mental Health and Mental Retardation Center, Carbondale, Pennsylvania.

5

Dance / Movement Therapy

It has become a commonplace that emotional states and mental problems manifest themselves in and through the body. We may literally blush with shame, snort with anger, frown in concentration, stare in amazement, gulp with surprise, pale with fright, retch with loathing, tremble with fear, and quiver with anticipation. We are all familiar with the obvious forms of psychosomatic expression: impotence, stuttering, allergies, hysterical blindness and paralysis, headaches, indigestion, asthma. Our language is studded with acknowledgments of this relationship: we have "gut reactions" to those we "can't stomach"; their ideas "stick in our craws" and may even make us "sick to our stomachs."

The young field of dance/movement therapy* is based on the growing realization that the psychosomatic relationship works both ways; it is equally a somatopsychic one. That strange genius

157

Wilhelm Reich observed that physical tensions invariably accompany mental tensions. He concluded that muscular tension and emotional repression are parallel symptoms of the same problem. Reich contended that the rigidity of the musculature is the somatic side of repression. In fact, he insisted, the body's failure to let go of tension is the basis for continuing states of repression. Reich wrote that mental and physical rigidities

> are not mutual expressions of one another, but form a unitary function.
> . . . Every neurotic is muscularly dystonic, and every cure is directly
> reflected in a change of muscular habitus [body stance and constitution].
> . . . Chronic muscular hypertension represents inhibition of every kind of
> excitation, of pleasure, anxiety and hatred alike. It is as if the inhibition
> of the vital functions (libido, anxiety, destruction) took place by way of
> the formation of a muscular armor around the center of the biological
> person. . . . . The antithetical relationship is clear; the physiological be-
> havior determines the psychic behavior and vice versa.[1]

As we have seen, however, the dichotomy between mind and body persists in the Western world. The view prevails that the mind represents the cognitive and the rational, the body the emotional, and that verbal language is the expression of the former, and non-verbal language of the latter. This view is still the traditional assumption in most psychotherapies, from which flows the conviction that none but verbal therapies can be useful in the treatment of mental disorders. It is only in recent years that the nonverbal therapies have begun to find some acceptance in the field of mental health.

As in the case of music therapy, the use of dance therapy can be traced to the influx of mental patients in hospitals during and after World War II. Dance therapist — educator Claire Schmais traces the emergence of dance therapy to the fact that individual psychoanalysis, based as it is on lengthy explorations into childhood traumas, was simply not capable of dealing with the large numbers of patients who were pouring into hospital mental wards.[2] Marian Chace, generally conceded to be the founder of modern dance therapy, writes: "In June of 1942 I started at Saint Elizabeth's Hospital

*The terms "dance therapy" and "movement therapy" are some-
times used interchangeably, but are frequently differentiated according
to the training, experience, and philosophies of the practitioners using
them. In its official communications, and in its definition of the field,
the American Dance Therapy Association uses the term "dance therapy."
However, because of semantic and ideological differences within the practice, the term "dance/movement therapy" has become popular as a broad
blanket name for the field.

with a dance program. We still did not call it dance therapy. We spoke of it only as dance for communication."[3]

In the fall of 1964, a small group of dance therapists who had trained with Chace met in Washington to discuss the formation of an association of dance therapists, and in 1966, a group of seventy-three charter members founded the American Dance Therapy Association (ADTA).[4] The official definition of dance therapy of the ADTA is, in part:

> Dance therapy is the psychotherapeutic use of movement as a process which furthers the emotional and physical integration of the individual.
>
> Dance therapists work with individuals who require special services because of behavioral, learning, perceptual and/or physical disorders. Dance therapy is used in the treatment, rehabilitation and education of the emotionally disturbed, physically handicapped, neurologically impaired and the socially deprived.

THE RESEARCH BASE

A central principle underlying the practice of dance/movement therapy is that *all* of our thoughts and emotions are inextricably interwoven with physical movement. This interrelationship has long been noted by observers and investigators. In his book, *The Expression of the Emotions in Man and Animals*, Charles Darwin dwelt at length on it. When a man struggles with an idea, Darwin noted, he may scratch his head, as though to relieve a physical irritation.[5] He concluded that the organism acts as a whole and performs the physical equivalent of mental operations.

More recently, cognitive and developmental psychologists like Jean Piaget and Jerome S. Bruner have underlined the role of the body in intellectual development. They agree that an individual proceeds through a hierarchical sequence of developmental stages, from the sensorimotor through the operational (Piaget's term for image making) to the symbolic.[6] Piaget contends that even in the later stages of development, thought is often *enactive*, involving internal imitation, and manifested by body movements and muscular tensions. These movements and tensions, Piaget says, actually represent mental symbolism.[7]

But accumulating evidence suggests that body movements not only reflect thought processes, they help create them. Many of us have experienced dreams that help us to interpret what is happening to our bodies during sleep; intricate plots are shaped instantaneously to explain itches or numbness, sensations of falling, or the dim sound of a bell ringing. Neurophysiobiologist Ernst Gellhorn points out that emotions, as well as thoughts, are shaped by the body. "Emotional behavior can be controlled via the somatic system," he contends, "or, to express it differently, . . . emotions can be controlled by willed action of the musculature."[8] A small but growing body of experimental and clinical evidence has been developing to support this view. Interestingly, most of these research data seem to come from fields outside of dance/movement therapy itself.

Edmund Jacobson, who developed a well-known system of "progressive relaxation," reported as far back as 1938 that his highly trained subjects found it impossible to retain emotions when they were in a state of complete physical relaxation. He suggested then that "an essential part of mental and emotional activities consists of neuromuscular patterns; the latter are not just 'expressions' of emotion."[9] Jacobson's later research demonstrates that every mental act, including perception, involves specifically patterned activity of the neuromuscular system.[10]

A good deal of solid and respectable research has seriously eroded the Western propensity to view humans in simple dichotomies — mind-body, willed-involuntary, inner-outer. Perhaps most dramatic has been the work of the pioneers in biofeedback — scientists like Neal Miller of Rockefeller University. Their research findings lend authoritative support to many of the concepts underlying the ancient Eastern view of humans as holistic organisms. Miller's work demonstrates that it is entirely possible, within the context of the Western scientific tradition, for humans to train and control not only their minds and the "voluntary" nervous and muscular systems, but the "autonomic," or reflex, system that had long been deemed beyond the reach of human will. Moreover, changes in one part of the organism invariably are accompanied by changes in other parts of the organism, a phenomenon that is highly supportive of a holistic view of body-mind.

Biofeedback has attracted the attention of diverse elements in the fields of mental and physical health. To humanists, biofeedback lends scientific respectability to concepts that, for the most part, had been intuitively derived. Moreover, the results of biofeedback research appear to provide some implicit support for the existence of mental states, such as consciousness, and for such concepts as volition that had previously been deemed inaccessible to scientific probing. Paradoxically, behaviorists tend to view biofeedback as a bolster to the behaviorist approach. The biofeedback signals are reinforcers of appropriate behavior. (The outstanding researchers in biofeedback tend to be behaviorists, although some, like Neal Miller, have taken issue with B. F. Skinner over the existence of "internal" stimuli.)

While biofeedback has captured the imagination of the public because of its obvious practicality in body-mind training, a series of discoveries have reinforced the holistic view of the human in another direction; research has added dimension to the idea that the body, as well as the mind, can learn and remember cognitively and affectively. As far back as the 1920s, neurosurgeons had discovered that electrical stimulation of parts of the brain could bring back vividly many forgotten scenes from the past and could evoke powerful emotions.[11] While the brain is obviously part of the human body, it is generally viewed as the repository of the mind, so the discovery did little to disturb the commonsense view that the memory and the emotions live up in the head.

In the 1960s, however, a number of interesting findings shook this conventional view. Ida Rolf, a biochemist who had turned to body therapy, developed an approach that she called *structural integration*, popularly known as "rolfing." In the course of her work, which involved manipulation of the muscles, Rolf found that pressures on particular muscles would often stimulate memories, sensations, and emotions.[12] Wilhelm Reich, who had earlier had similar experiences, had hypothesized that memories and emotions are stored in the muscles as well as in the brain.

Much of the modern research base for the field is derived from the relatively young field of *kinesics*, the science of body-behavioral communication, frequently popularized as "body language." Ray L. Birdwhistell, a pioneer in the field, is an anthropologist whose early field work raised questions in his mind about the adequacy of either a verbal communication or an imitation theory of socialization within a culture. Investigation convinced him that the bulk of human communication may be nonverbal. Speech itself, he contends, is much more than combinations of words; the real substance of socially organized interpersonal behavior is expressed in sounds, intonations, silences, postures, and gestures.[13]

To be accepted as a member of a society, contends Birdwhistell, an individual must master the communications system of that society — verbal and nonverbal. Our definition of sanity is based on a social view; it involves behavior that is both appropriate and predictable. We *can* cope with inappropriate behavior, according to Birdwhistell, but only if we can anticipate it; social behavior and communication that is both inappropriate and unpredictable is defined as insanity. "Undiagnosed unpredictability in others," he writes, "leaves us with doubts about ourselves. So the definition of others as insane permits us to deal with them."

But "insane" behavior is not as chaotic or disordered as we would like to believe. The schizophrenic merely has a different and — to most of us — an inappropriate system of communication. In addition, the emotionally disturbed seem to have a greater capacity for misinterpreting the behavior of others and "when ill, they do not seem to have the same ability to modify their behavior when it is offensive or misunderstood."[14]

Much of the research in kinesics relies on technology for recording and analyzing communication. William S. Condon, a psychologist then working at the University of Pittsburgh, analyzed hundreds of sound films, frame by frame, and found a surprisingly ordered and rhythmical physical element in speech itself. Condon confirmed relationships that had been noted years earlier between the body movements of a speaker and his or her speech patterns, a relationship known as *self-synchrony*. The body as a whole seems constantly to be undergoing change during the process of speech.[15]

Continued analysis of films led to a startling discovery. In addition to the self-synchrony of a speaker, Condon and others found, changes occur in the body movements of listeners. Moreover, these body changes are surprisingly correlated with the movements of the speaker, in a pattern that has come to be known as *interactional synchrony*. This phenomenon occurs consistently and cuts across cultures; among the films analyzed were communications among !Kung bushmen, Eskimos, and Mayan Indians. The intricate patterns of relationships often occur within periods of a single frame ($1/24$ of a second). Body changes of speaker and listener — leaning forward, moving arms or legs or torso, blinking eyes — tend to speed up and slow down together or in proportionate speeds "like puppets being moved by the same set of strings."[16]

Condon was struck by the order and grace of these movements, many of them imperceptible to the unaided eye, and repeatedly remarks on the participant and inherent "dancelike" quality of interaction. These findings, Condon told an audience of dance therapists in 1968, are of major significance for dance/movement therapy, which "would seem to be admirably suited to initiate or re-initiate communication. Moving together in harmony *is* communication."[17]

Later research underlines the rhythmic quality in interactional synchrony. Even unseen rhythmic actions — as when someone taps a foot or swings a leg behind a desk — are picked up in a listener's body when the individuals are in rapport. Many observers find an analogy in musical resonance (the vibrations from one instrument will induce another to resonate in the same pitch) and go so far as to suggest that the transfer of vibrations, or "resonances," between people involves a real transfer of energy as well as a subconscious "reading" of body movement.[18] It is significant that emotional disorder often leads to a loss of interactional synchrony and even of self-synchrony.

Recent studies show that the synchronous social development of humans begins at a surprisingly early age. Condon and Louis W. Sander, in the course of careful observations at Boston University Medical Center, found that as early as the first day of life, the human infant moves "in precise and sustained segments of movement that are synchronous with the articulated structure of human speech."[19] The investigators hypothesize that infants are active participants in human interaction and that they internalize and entrain millions of repetitions of linguistic forms long before they later use them in speaking.

The early development of such interactional behaviors is of particular interest to those who work in early child development. Child psychiatrist Judith S. Kestenberg has found that infants and mothers engage in reciprocal "holding" patterns, in which not only does the mother hold the child, but the child "holds" the mother as well, by its weight distribution, its effort flow, and its shaping patterns. Through mutual accommodation, mother and child learn to trust each other. Says Kestenberg: "The *trustworthy* baby does not lean on the mother so heavily that she cannot breathe in comfort, nor does the *trustworthy* mother hold him in a rigid embrace which interferes with his respiration. The same is true of shape-flow rhythms."[20]

Kestenberg's observations coincide with findings of those in kinesics research, who remark on the frequency with which schizophrenic mothers may communicate "double messages" to their infants in the course of handling them and on the development by such infants of dyssynchronous postures and movements.[21] Kestenberg writes: "It becomes very apparent to the observer of infants that early positions and directions imposed upon the infant can become embedded in individual body attitudes."[22] The significance of such study seems to lie in the potential the findings offer for preventive as well as for therapeutic work.

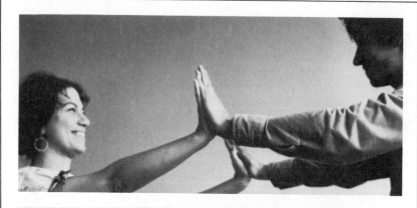

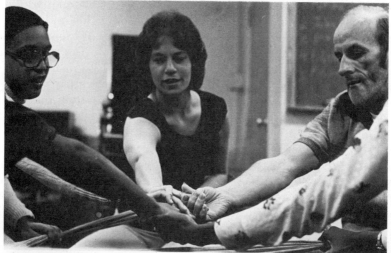

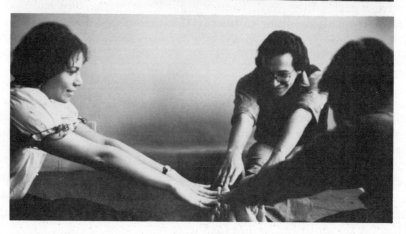

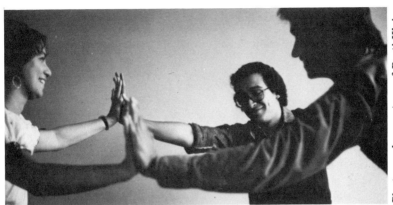

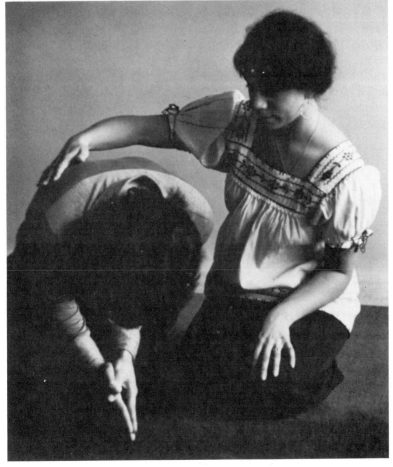

DANCE/MOVEMENT
IN DIAGNOSIS

It is much easier for an individual to conceal his or her feelings and thoughts in verbal communication than it is in movement. Unlike verbal language, the language of the body never ceases, even in repose. It betrays our innermost thoughts. In his essay, "Fragment of an Analysis of a Case of Hysteria," Freud wrote: "He that has eyes to see and ears to hear may convince himself that no mortal can keep a secret. If his lips are silent, he chatters with his fingertips; betrayal oozes out of him at every pore."[23]

This physical language, difficult to control at best and partly beyond deliberate control, enables dance/movement therapists to probe beneath the surface. Warren Lamb, a long-time student of human movement, says: "While we cannot observe mental behavior (unless we claim to be mind readers) we can accurately observe physical behavior, i.e., what the body and the parts of the body are doing."[24] And increasingly, observers have come to believe that when verbal messages and those sent by the body contradict each other, the movement is the more accurate messenger.[25]

Dance/movement focuses on that constant betrayer of the inner self, the human body, as do the "body therapies." Unlike some of the body therapies, however, dance/movement is based on the idea that what is *most* significant about the body is not physique or position, but movement. "To observe behavior," says Warren Lamb, "means to observe variation. The position itself is of no interest; we want to know how the person got into it."[26]

Observing and classifying movement can be done in many ways. Like developmentalist Arnold Gesell, we can focus on *function*, or the use of movement to perform specific tasks.[27] We can look for *tensions*, as did Wilhelm Reich.[28] We can focus on the symbolic use of *position* and *direction*,[29] or of *posture* and *gesture*.[30] Dance/movement therapy makes use of all of these classification systems to some extent. But, while the evidence is continual and continuous, it is fleeting, and the therapist often must record the shapes, tensions, directions, and movement patterns for diagnosis. While the use of film or videotape may be helpful in preserving the movement for review, it is limited in its value for *analysis*.

Several descriptive, analytical systems have been developed for coding, recording, and analyzing movement. The two that are best known are *Labanotation*, a system created by Rudolf Laban for recording movement patterns and weight distribution,[31] and *Effort/ Shape*, an outgrowth and an extension of Laban's system, designed

166

specifically to focus on tensions, efforts, and shapes.[32] Labanotation is concerned with the quantitative elements of movement (the "what") and has become a standard notation system in dance choreography. Effort/shape deals with the qualitative aspects of movement (the "how") and is therefore more useful in dance/movement therapy diagnosis. (See *A Tool of the Trade*, p. 189.)

A number of studies show that the observations of trained effort/shape analysts correlate well with data about body tensions that are measured electrically or mechanically. One study, for example, reports a clear concurrence between the observations of five observers and the recorded measurements on electromyographical (EMG) activity from a patient's muscles.[33]

It might seem difficult to record and analyze movement patterns—and it is. It takes years to train a competent effort/shape analyst. But two facts make the task less difficult than it might appear at first. Laban had early noted that an individual's movements seldom occur in isolation; they are expressed in paths and patterns that Laban called "trace forms."[34] In addition, observers have pointed out that these patterns are usually repeated by the same individual again and again.[35] As a result, the recorder need only identify the *modus operandi* for diagnosis, and this can emerge from scattered, brief notations.

Nevertheless, while the terminology of effort/shape is widely used among practitioners, the use of the notation system itself is less widespread. As we mentioned, proficiency in notation requires at least two years of intensive training. Moreover, it has been found that it is extremely difficult for a movement therapist simultaneously to conduct a movement session and record a client's movement patterns. As a result, a recent development is the distinction between notation and therapy and the growth of a separate category of effort/shape notator, who may be called in to help dance/movement therapists as the occasion arises.

Most therapists limit their analyses of clients to "movement assessments," rather than to psychological diagnoses. They will distinguish and note movement patterns and identify those that may themselves be revealing or "dysfunctional." The therapist may look for constricted movement, undue muscle tension, uncontrolled — or overcontrolled — movement. In addition, of course, the therapist will seek to learn more about feelings that accompany movement or that are expressed through movement.

Once the evidence is recorded, the diagnosis itself—if a psychological diagnosis is desired—is often undertaken in group consultations, in which groups of nonverbal therapists operate in teams with psychotherapists to pool their findings. Certain correlations may be noted between body patterns and traditional psychologically labeled disorders.[36] For example, one characteristic of psychotic behavior in general is behavior rigidity, an inability to switch from a stereotyped method of coping and a lack of creativity and adaptability.[37] Mental retardates typically display "motor impersistence"; their movements start and stop suddenly as the muscles go limp, and they tend to imitate movements rather than initiate them. Paradoxically, they also tend to "perseverate"—that is, to persist in simple activities long after normal individuals have given up in boredom. Schizophrenics, whose body image fantasies often center on the loss or destruction of the body boundaries, may have an unrealistic sense of the limits of their bodies and highly distorted images of their own bodies. Those who are generally characterized as obsessive-compulsives, on the other hand, often bear a strong sense of shame and guilt about their bodies; their movements may appear tense and rigid. The movements of a hysteric tend to be soft, sequential, agile. "The neurotic ego dominates the body," concluded Alexander Lowen, "the schizoid ego denies it, while the schizophrenic ego dissociates from it."[38]

Some attempts have been made to carry the diagnostic function of movement analysis to a one-to-one relationship between movement patterns and psychological traits. In one such study, taped intake interviews at a psychiatric outpatient clinic were later correlated with the tape of comments by a viewer behind a one-way mirror to whom the conversations were inaudible. A close correlation was reported between the diagnosis of the verbal psychotherapist and that of the movement analyst. Some of the specifics noted focused on basic gesture interpretations: rubbing or touching the nose was related to contempt, disgust, and negative feelings; finger-mouth contact with oral-erotic needs and gratification; self-rubbing with tension reduction; and picking, smoothing, and cleaning with compulsive traits.

Some actions, it was reported, expressed the same meaning as the concomitant verbal content: for example, the removal of eyeglasses suggested difficulty in facing or seeing problems. Some gestures did not appear on the surface to be related to verbal content, but turned out later to have anticipated subsequent amplifications. Some gestures betrayed thoughts and feelings that belied the words of the subject: a male patient who deftly manipulated a pencil throughout most of his interview, for example, lost control of the pencil and dropped it when he was claiming defensively that his work was 100-percent efficient.[39]

One study correlated expressive movement styles as described in effort/shape terms with personality characteristics ascertained through the use of a questionnaire. Among the findings: anxious individuals avoided "light" movements; "carefree, fun-loving" individuals showed a preference for "indirect" movement; and "adventurous" individuals preferred "strong" and "free" movements.[40] Similarly, Elaine V. Siegel, a movement therapist at the Center for Emotionally Disturbed Children in Suffolk County, New York, developed what she calls a "developmental outline" in which she has identified "symptomatic motility" as related to "nosological categories" for infants and children. For example, she describes symptoms of child schizophrenia in physical terms:

> Hyperactivity or catatonia. Body distortions with and without fantasy content. Bizarre gestures. Head rolling. Rocking. Fusion of hips and torso. Fusion of head, neck and torso. Toe walking. Tension around mouth and neck. Drooling. Biting. Dystonia. . . . Arhythmicity of breathing and speech. Ability at height of symbiosis to imitate others' rhythms totally.[41]

Childhood obsession-compulsion is described in terms of "general body tension, particularly around sphincter and buttocks," "erect, rigid posture," "slackness of all muscles," and "highly structured use of rhythms." Movement symptoms of hysteria include "diffuse gestures," "restricted pelvic swing," and "shallow breathing patterns."[42]

Most observers in the field seem to be wary of such facile pairings of symptomatic manifestation and psychological diagnostic labeling. Claire Schmais is much more cautious, reporting only that "the movements [of most psychotics] tend to be distorted, fragmented, reduced dynamically, limited spatially and often inappropriate. . . . They often are synchronous neither with self nor with others."[43] Child psychiatrist Judith S. Kestenberg, who correlates much of her movement analysis with the psychoanalytic maturation development stages of Anna Freud, makes it quite clear that she does not attempt a one-to-one relationship of physical movement and psychological trait.[44]

Indeed, some dance/movement therapists resist the conversion of movement observations into psychological terms, on the ground that movement analysis and movement therapy alone should be enough, since the body-mind relationship works both ways. A number of calls have gone forth to dance/movement therapists to develop their own classification systems, rather than to borrow categories and labels from the fields of psychology and psychiatry. Dance/movement, says Irmgard Bartenieff, a leader in movement analysis and notation, "should fully develop its own fundamentals and terminology before entering the field of science in order that it not yield too readily to the tendency to borrow terms from psychiatry, psychology or physiology in the attempt to make itself acceptable as a therapeutic tool."[45]

Dance therapists have been urged to develop their own categories and their own language of movement, as well as their own research programs in movement problems, rather than in movement as a manifestation of psychological problems. Harris Chaiklin warns that "if dance therapy does not develop its own knowledge base and devise ways to apply this systematically to practice, it will end as a minor adjunctive technique."[46]

THE THERAPEUTIC USE
OF DANCE/MOVEMENT

A kaleidoscope of reports from everywhere testifies to the therapeutic use of dance/movement. A four-year-old victim of congenital hemiplegia is taught to creep on all fours, to perform simple body movements—and his speech improves.[47] A depressed patient who is assigned to a dance therapy session reports that afterward he can speak more freely with his psychotherapist.[48] A forty-year-old woman patient in a mental health day treatment center sits withdrawn while a group performs simple *kolos*—Macedonian circle dances—until she succumbs to "behavioral contagion" and joins the circle; she moves rhythmically, arm-in-arm with others. Clinic workers report that for the rest of the day she talks with others, something that had been rare before.[49]

At the Easter Seal Center in Rockville, Maryland, preschool children with language handicaps are helped to expand their horizons through the use of body movement, which provides creative outlets for personality growth—and their speech becomes less garbled.[50] A hospitalized schizophrenic young woman in a long-range movement therapy program demonstrates an increasing interaction with the dance therapist; her psychotherapist reports increased and warmer contacts with him, with other staff and patients, and with visitors.[51]

Such experiences reflect the growing recognition in mental health that movement is not merely a manifestation of personality but is actually a part of personality. Movement and stance express an individual's emotional state, but they also help to shape it. For example, subjects under hypnosis cannot feel emotions that are inconsistent with their physical postures or body stances.[52] And Paul Schilder writes: "When there is a specific motor sequence it changes the inner situation and attitudes and even provokes a phantasy situation which fits the muscular sequence."[53]

Alexander Lowen goes so far as to insist that the cure of many psychoses *must* involve some body change:

> The conflict between the ego and the body produces a split in the personality which affects all aspects of an individual's existence and behavior. . . . The split cannot be resolved without improving the condition of the body. Breathing must be deepened, motility increased, and feelings evoked if the body is to become more alive and its reality is to govern the ego images.[54]

All dance/movement therapists approach the "psychoorganism" (a recently coined term that is popular, especially in humanist circles) through the body, but there are wide variations in goals and methods. Further, many factors influence the specifics of a dance/movement therapy program. Patient populations range from articulate and sociable alcoholic outpatients to severely regressed hospitalized psychotics. The philosophic and theoretical orientation of the institution or the psychotherapist with whom a dance/movement therapist works may be Freudian, Jungian, Adlerian, behavioristic, or gestalt. Moreover, the therapist may choose to work on a one-to-one basis to elicit "authentic" movement or in groups to encourage socialization. She (most dance/movement therapists are women) may prefer to use music to prompt movement response and stimulate emotion (as did Marian Chace), or she may prefer silence to encourage authentic expression.

More important than the psychological or philosophical orientation of the therapist, in shaping the nature of the therapy encounter, is the nature of the relationship between the patient and the therapist; the therapist must constantly be sensitive to the momentary needs of the patient and must, in Theodor Reik's words, "listen with the third ear."

Probably the most important influence on the shape of the program is the long-range goals that the therapist has set, while the specifics of the individual session are determined by the functions on which the therapist concentrates. Functions do overlap, however, and few sessions are one-dimensional.

Body Awareness

At a very early age, an individual has developed a *muscle memory* —a stance and movement pattern to respond to external situations and to express emotions and feelings. (It should be noted that the term "muscle memory" has a very different meaning as it is used in some contexts; some who manipulate the body report, as does Ida Rolf, that pressures on muscles may trigger sensations, emotions, and deeply buried memories.) Much of the muscle pattern is rooted in the culture of the individual; southerners smile much more than northerners, for example.[55] Much of it, however, is idiosyncratic. The muscle memory of an individual may or may not be tuned to the environment productively; the movements may or may not be appropriate to external circumstances. The range of movements may be extensive or constricted. In a very real sense, the muscle memory is part of an individual's personality.

One very basic goal of dance/movement therapy may be the simple expansion of a movement vocabulary to increase the ability of an individual to express moods, attitudes, and ideas. Autistic children, for example, who have never developed a full range of interaction with their environments and who have not developed communicative speech, display virtually no evidence of interactional synchrony. Indeed, the movements of many psychotics often reveal an absence of synchrony between the parts of their own bodies. Stiff, contracted legs may belie limp hands; one eye may move while the other remains fixed.

Subjected to frame analysis, almost all films of pathological behavior cases have been found to be self-dyssynchronous.[56] Autistic children seem never to have formed coherent images of their own bodies; they seem unaware of persons as well—including their own parents. As infants, they fail to assume anticipatory positions when being picked up, and they fail to adjust their own bodies to those who hold them.[57] Movements tend to be disjointed, disconnected, unpredictable, and apparently purposeless.

It has been pointed out that "the self-image of the body is inseparable from the self-image of the personality and both reflects and affects that image,"[58] and Mitchell L. Dratman, a physician who has done a good deal of work with autistic children, says that without an accurate body image,

> the psychic structure necessary for symbolic representation of other things cannot be formed, since they depend on previous symbolization. Consequently, it is reasonable that the autistic child develops no words to form ideas so he cannot make the bridge from the concrete to the abstract.[59]

A basic function of dance/movement therapy, therefore, may be to help such individuals gain control over their own bodies and to develop accurate body images, which are indispensable for the building of the self-image that will permit the individual to see himself in relation to the world outside. The schizophrenic, who is often confused about the limits of his body and the way it relates to everything outside, may be helped to redefine his boundaries. The obsessive-compulsive, whose body limits are unduly constricted, and who bears a strong sense of guilt and shame about his body, may be helped to accept his body, to enjoy physical experiences, and to expand his movements.

For more sophisticated or less-disturbed patients, body discovery may focus on the recognition of tensions and constrictions, as well as on the development of body alignment and centering. Movement analysts are constantly impressed with the inability of most normal persons to recognize their own misalignments, which may be correlated with a host of physical and emotional problems. This body-awareness function seems to be a major focus of some of the humanistic therapies; unfortunately, many therapists who deal with body awareness are not trained movement therapists and may be poorly prepared and minimally competent to deal with physical aspects of body problems.

The term "coping" is often used in connection with the body-awareness function. Occasionally, a heightened awareness alone — of signals that the body is sending, or of movement possibilities of which we might previously have been unaware — may in itself help us to deal with a problem. But the assumption is usually unwarranted that the ability to *recognize* a problem can automatically be converted into the ability to *cope* with it. For example, an individual may be made aware that a tightening of the neck muscles is a signal of tension, but he or she may not know how to deal with the problems that trigger the signal, or even how to relieve the tension itself. So unless the therapist can help the patient to cope at least with the physical problem, the awareness alone may be of limited value.

Since tension invariably has both its mental and physical manifestations, a basic principle in dance/movement therapy is that relief in one aspect of the problem will mean relief in the other. The therapist may use a number of techniques for relief when the signal is recognized. For example, behaviorist researchers have verified the incompatibility of certain activities (reciprocal inhibition), and a therapist may teach a patient the principles of deep breathing or progressive relaxation when he or she recognizes the onset of the physical tension that accompanies mental anxiety.

Catharsis

Sometimes referred to as *release* or *discharge*, this function is based on the recognition that body activity can help an individual to "let go" of a suppressed emotion. The human organism often resorts to "self-catharsis," as when a disturbed individual vomits to "get rid" of a distressing thought or memory. We are often unable — literally — to "swallow" disturbing ideas. A common application of the cathartic function of movement is the pummeling of a pillow or a wall in a symbolic aggression.

In many cases, individuals are inhibited in their verbal expression of anger or anxiety and may feel safer "acting out" their emotions. Because dance is often associated with exhibition, patients may find it an acceptable medium in which to express — and confront — their own otherwise suppressed exhibitionistic and narcissistic tendencies. For many of the early years of dance therapy, its primary function had been considered catharsis, or "emotional release." A traditional activity in groups led by Marian Chace was "shaking off everything"; participants would kick their pressures into the center of the circle for mass destruction.[60]

Patients in dance/movement therapy may express their hidden impulses, conflicts, feelings, and confusions in a variety of ways. Writing of the myriad of expressions, dance therapy pioneer Trudi Schoop described a "tango of hate," in which the patient's movements began with little stamps, followed by brusque turns, lashing arms, and ended with the patient walking in ever-closing inward spirals until he stood at the center in a world of his own.[61] A dance therapist in a situation in which patient populations may be transient and inhibited may choose to use patterned set dances as a nonthreatening introduction to cathartic movement; a patient may engage in Rumanian folk dances that call for vigorous foot stamping, when he is not yet ready to express his own violent — and frightening — emotions in "authentic" movement, or expose his private and guarded secrets to others.

By and large, the cathartic function of dance/movement therapy is not supported enthusiastically by Freudian psychoanalysts, who appear reluctant to see patients' tensions and anxieties reduced. Dance therapy's cathartic function, they believe, reduces the commitment of a patient to psychoanalysis. This view is consistent with Freud's own rejection of catharsis in therapy. Freud stated that permanent changes in personality could be brought about only "as far as possible under privation — in a state of abstinence," and that "the patient must have unfulfilled wishes in abundance."[62] Psychoanalyst Reuben Fine writes that "Freud's early emphasis on catharsis has been almost entirely superseded by his later emphasis on insight. . . . Catharsis may offer some immediate relief to some patients, but it never plays a major role in the contemporary psychoanalytic treatment process."[63] Moreover, many psychoanalysts fear that, in the patient-therapist relationship, the cathartic function may degenerate into fantasy indulgence and serve as catharsis only in the sense of "transference cures" that last only as long as an idealized therapist-patient relationship lasts.

As in art therapy, some dance/movement therapists believe that cathartic release is itself healing. Many practitioners, however, seem to agree that exposure alone is not enough. "Once a person's feelings of conflict have been brought into the body," writes Trudi Schoop, "improvisation has served its main purpose. There's no point in going on and on with it, for no matter how many times the body 'admits' to a feeling, it will continue to express it in the same manner, over and over."[64] While expression of an emotion or a problem may serve a cathartic function of relief, eventually the deep-seated conflicts and confusions will again accumulate. Mere discharges, Schoop contends, "can become a mindless circle, a kind of self-indulgence. There will be no change in the problem itself. Something constructive has to be done about it."[65]

Humanists tend to be more favorably disposed toward the cathartic function. John Heider, who had directed human potential programs at Esalen Institute, writes in *The Journal of Humanistic Psychology* that a cathartic release of pent-up emotions or tensions is frequently followed by an unusual, "even ecstatic" sense of well-being. "In this postcathartic state," Heider contends, "conditions for healing, growth, and transcendence exist to an unusual degree; psychosomatic symptoms fall away, insights into personal behavior come easily and naturally, and a transcendent sense of union with cosmic order is common."[66]

Whether or not they accept the idea that catharsis can lead to "transcendence," many dance/movement therapists agree that physical release can lead to a condition of receptivity to therapy, or growth, or self-awareness. In the later stages of treatment, it is also generally agreed, movement and cognitive work must be viewed as complementary. This "two-factor" approach will be discussed in greater depth in a later section.

Interpersonal Communication

Researchers in kinesics believe that the bulk of human communication is nonverbal. To the extent that, as William Condon put it, "movement *is* communication," increasing an individual's choices in movement enlarges that individual's ability to understand and be understood by others.

Frequently, movement is one of the few ways of establishing contact with patients who may be, in Marian Chace's words, "locked in a world of silence." Autistic children may first be approached on their own primitive levels of movement, in the hope of establishing the interactional synchrony that is essential to emotional relationships with other humans. A standard technique is "mirroring," in which the therapist incorporates the child's rhythms and gestures into her own movement patterns. Describing the technique, body-movement therapist Beth Kalish — who has specialized in movement work with autistic children — stresses the delicate balance that is needed: too much mirroring may cause the child to withdraw even more, and too little will fail to establish contact.[67] Mirroring (not mimicking) may establish the basis for the social bonding that the autistic child has never experienced, and it may help him or her to establish a body image.

An enlarged movement vocabulary not only helps the patient to express emerging impulses and feelings, but it enables him or her to interpret more accurately the signals of others. The hysteric, to whom a handshake may be a sexual overture, the paranoid schizophrenic, to whom it may be an assault, the obsessive-neurotic, to whom it may be a challenge,[68] learn to recognize and differentiate the messages of nonverbal communication. What Scheflen calls "metasignals" or "qualifying signals" help individuals to recognize when apparently hostile or seductive communications are not to be taken seriously.[69]

The stylized and stereotyped movements of folk dances may be used to help patients recognize these disclaimers. Moreover, the group identity, the sharing with others, may be the first step toward the development of an expanded nonverbal and finally verbal communication. Such "set" dances are frequently performed in circles, the symbol of unity in Jungian and much of humanistic therapy, and are most appropriate in short-term treatment settings, where intensive "authentic" movement experiences are inhibited by large numbers and limited patient-therapist contact. (See *A Tool of the Trade*, p. 194.)

The group experience itself can provide the feedback that enables a patient to distinguish between fantasy and reality. Trudi Schoop describes Alice, who wept bitterly because "they want to separate me from my friends on Venus." After Alice had described the activities and the music on Venus, Schoop and a group of patients filled the room with sounds of bells, triangles, and gongs to accompany a floating dance. "Rarely have I seen a stage director directing his group so confidently, or performers who could so easily identify with his images," Schoop writes.[70]

Whatever the content of a patient's delusion, Schoop contends, acting it out in a group has three therapeutic results:[71]

1. The patient has exposed his delusion, and, to the extent that he has shared it with others, he has weakened its power to control his existence.
2. The patient is better able to contrast reality with delusion. (Alice knew that she was in a hospital studio, not on Venus, "and that the one who kissed her was good old Betty, not Clandestine." But if her friends on earth could respond to her in much the same way as her friends on Venus, perhaps reality was not so bad.)
3. Because the patient is forced to deal with fantasy and reality, "he is led toward the discovery of the healthy balance" between the imaginary and the mundane. ("So I feel," says Schoop, "that rather than suppressing the fantasy of a psychotic individual, we should fly with him for a while, then descend with him for a soft landing on this earth.")

Among the most significant developments in the study of the body as social communicator is the increasing recognition that cultural mores, as well as "psychological" experiences, leave imprints on an individual's movement patterns and ways of dealing with the environment. In the behavioral sciences, there are two ways of looking at "body language." One is the "psychological" view that the body mainly communicates expressions of internal feelings — that we can "read" an individual's feelings by observing his or her posture, gestures, movement patterns. The other position, derived from such disciplines as anthropology and ethology (a science that focuses on the relationships between organisms and their environments), views body position and movement in terms of social functions and processes. For example, an observer might ask, What role does such activity play in controlling the behavior of others?

Albert Scheflen, an authority in kinesics, has had extensive experience in both ways of looking at body behavior. He had long been a practicing psychoanalyst before he turned to the intensive study of kinesics and language in relation to culture and social organization. In the preface to the book *Body Language and Social Order* that he wrote with his wife Alice, he says:

In the last few years a broad interest in body language has developed out-side the formal sciences of man. Unfortunately the interest has taken a largely psychological slant, such that body behaviors are merely given psychodynamic meanings. Thus, we are led to believe that crossing the legs "means" that one fears castration or that a particular facial expression or touch "means" that one loves his mother or the like. Such simplistic views ignore twenty years of research, a systems revolution in modern thought, the social, economic and political contexts of human behavior and the cultural differences in American society.[72]

Middle-class Americans, Scheflen observes, tend toward this kind of oversimplification, often ignoring the determining role of cultural, social, economic, and political processes in human affairs. Virtually every major scholar in kinesics has emphasized the role of culture and environment in shaping "body language." Birdwhistell called his major book *Kinesics and Context* to emphasize the point that body language has meaning only in a social and cultural environ-ment. Professionals in the various psychotherapies and in the emerg-ing nonverbal therapies are likely to fall victim to the one-dimensional oversimplifications mainly because of their tendency to view patients in terms of psychological categories.

A therapist who is ignorant of, or heedless of, a patient's cultural background and of the nuances of social communication in the patient's environment may make serious errors in diagnosis or in treatment. A patient may fail to maintain eye contact because of personal "psychological" problems. Or he or she may have been brought up in a culture in which one does not make eye contact with strangers: in some minority cultures in America, maintaining eye contact is a sign of hostility or aggression. Similarly, the therapist who insists that patients touch each other, in the naive belief that touching is a universal gesture of rapport, may be creating a highly uncomfortable, or even a threatening, environment for the patient in whose culture strangers do not touch, or in which individuals need considerable personal "body space."

Sensitive dance/movement therapists are cautious enough in their approach to clients to ease into a relationship, and they may avoid such errors intuitively. Gimmick therapists, committed to a technique rather than to a relationship, are likely to be the major offenders.

Restructuring

The body therapies are based on the idea that producing changes in the body on a neuromuscular level will produce not only physical, but mental, changes. Most of them derive from the theories of Wilhelm Reich, who contended that life experiences are locked into the muscles and the skeletal structure. For example, premature toilet training might stimulate resistance through muscle spasms in the pelvic area — a pattern that would persist into adulthood, distorting posture, constricting blood vessels, and preventing the flow of energy into the lower part of the body. Reich's heresy was disavowed by traditional psychoanalysts, but it formed the basis for the growing number of body therapies. A slowly developing pool of empirical data has developed in recent years that supports at least some elements of Reich's theories; much of it comes from the work of researchers in biofeedback.

Most of the body therapies involve physical restructuring, either through external manipulation or postural training. Among the best known of these are Ida Rolf's *structural integration*, commonly called "rolfing," in which the body's structure is "realigned" for optimum posture and flexibility; Alexander Lowen's *bioenergetics*, which attempts to release neuromuscular blocks in order to permit energy and feelings to flow through the body; the *Alexander Technique*, which seeks to correct the relationship between head, neck, and torso; and the method of Moshe Feldenkrais, whose therapy seeks to "unlock" constrictions, especially in the pelvic area. To the degree that they seek to create major postural change, some of the exotic imports, like *Yoga, Aikido,* and *T'ai chi,* may be classified as restructuring approaches.

The notion of external manipulation has not found favor among dance/movement therapists, most of whom believe that basic change can result only from conscious — or at least willed — movement work. Some of the techniques and patterns of the Eastern movement and postural training programs have been incorporated by some humanistically inclined therapists and some who work with specific clients, such as the elderly, for whom slow, repetitive, or routinized movements may be important. With such groups, however, the restructuring function may not be of primary importance. For the most part, restructuring cannot be considered a major function of dance/movement therapy.

Communicating with the Unconscious

In the psychoanalytic view, which dominates dance/movement therapy, our movements help project our preverbal and undifferentiated feelings into the level of consciousness. The movements of the body, therefore, bring to the surface the repressed emotions, the instinctual demands, and the "unfinished business" that we have tried to bury. The symbolic acting out inherent in improvised "authentic" body movements facilitates the emergence of hidden impulses, memories, and emotions.

As in art therapy, some practitioners believe that this "consciousness-raising" is itself therapeutic. However, many, if not most, therapists think that the postures, gestures, tensions, and sensations must be identified, recognized, and translated, and the emotions that have been aroused must be interpreted verbally.

In one series of imaginative experiments, it was found that it was possible to lead subjects who were "experiencing" precisely the same chemically induced state of physiological arousal to think that they were feeling angry or euphoric or otherwise emotionally affected.[73] Apparently, physiological arousal alone is ambiguous and may be subject to misinterpretation unless an opportunity is provided to discuss, differentiate, and label the surfaced feelings. There seems to be a general agreement that all movement work should include or be supplemented by verbal cognitive work.

Many dance/movement therapists work in teams with psychotherapists, who help the patient to sort out and identify the feelings that emerge from the movement experiences. This team approach is common in hospitals and clinics. Growing numbers of movement therapists, however, have been entering the field from the disciplines of psychology and psychotherapy, rather than from dance, from which the practice derived.* Many of these psychologically based therapists tend to reject not only the label of dance therapist, but even that of movement therapist, preferring to call themselves movement psychotherapists. They tend to think of themselves as primary, rather than adjunctive, therapists, and they combine experiential and verbal therapy in their own sessions.

---

*Ostensibly, training in dance therapy (as it is officially called by the ADTA) spans the two fields. As a prerequisite for a graduate program in dance therapy, the ADTA recommends a degree in dance *or* psychology "and extensive dance training in technique, theory, improvisation, pedagogy, and choreography." The master's degree program that is recommended includes group dynamics, psychology of personality, abnormal psychology, theory of individual and group psychotherapy, applied anatomy, and kinesiology. In actuality, those who enter the field with a dance background may, in fact, have had "extensive" dance training — often from childhood. On the other hand, those who come to the program with degrees in psychology sometimes view the field as a specialized form of psychotherapy, and such individuals may see the dance courses they take as supplemental. So the difference is primarily one of background experiences, orientation, and interest.

CURRENT ISSUES IN
DANCE/MOVEMENT THERAPY

The role of dance/movement therapy in mental health is circumscribed by the attitude of psychotherapists. For the most part, psychotherapists are indifferent to the nonverbal therapies. In a 1976 publication called *The Therapist's Handbook*, for example, there is not a single index listing under art, music, dance or movement. The only section of the book devoted to "somatic therapies" is limited to a discussion of electric convulsive therapy.[74] As we have noted, many psychoanalytically oriented therapists are suspicious of, if not hostile to, the cathartic function, and are generally unenthusiastic about the efficacy of any but predominantly verbal techniques in the integrative function of reconciling the conscious and the unconscious. Many Freudians see dance/movement therapy as an adjunctive therapy whose only real value is as an aid in diagnosis.

However, there have been real contributions to the field by some Freudian analysts as well as by some in other psychoanalytic groups, especially those who subscribe to the theories of Jung, Sullivan, and Reich (whom many psychoanalysts consider an apostate, a "defrocked" analyst). Reich's views on muscular armor, of course, coincide with the goal of reducing muscular tensions as a prerequisite for movement for expression or integration. A number of studies have found that engaging patients in movement patterns specifically designed to free the chronically rigid areas allows for the expression of repressed emotions.[75] For the most part, dance/ movement therapists tend to view the reduction in muscular tension less as an end in itself than as a precondition for more meaningful therapeutic work.

Jungian psychoanalysis, which has given so much support to art therapy, is also supportive of the use of movement as a means of maintaining a dialogue with the unconscious. Because of the nonliteral nature of so much that is creative, Jungian dance therapists — with the support of Jungian analysts — view the creative act as a symbolic expression of deep feelings, especially when words fail — as they do so frequently among the mentally disturbed. Moreover, to Jungians, the ability to create is in itself an indication of individuation.

A major characteristic of psychotic behavior is its rigidity, marked by imitation, repetition, and stereotyped activities. The artistic experience, which Jung called "active imagination," is a key to creativity, to getting outside of the ego, so that the unconscious, along with the conscious, can be expressed. Mary Whitehouse, a Jungian dance therapist, believes that "the activated unconscious" always seeks expression, and that body movement is direct, in contrast with the indirect expression that obtains in many therapies. "I discovered," she writes, "that I worked directly with the unconscious when I worked with the body."[76] Some Jungians see idiosyncratic movement as the somatic representation of what Jung called the *shadow* — the unknown or darker side of personality — whose recognition is necessary for self-knowledge and wholeness.[77]

Similarly, dance therapists who have been influenced by Sullivan's interpersonal theory of personality enjoy the support of Sullivanian psychotherapists, who see dance therapy as a medium for resocialization. Therapist and patient can make contact, first in the *parataxic* mode (in which things occur together accidentally), and then in the *syntaxic* mode (which occurs when meaning is shared).[78] Because the dance or movement experience involves active participation with others, it is deemed to be therapeutic, as well as diagnostic.

The relationship between dance/movement therapy and humanism involves something of a paradox. Dance therapy and humanism share a common view of the holistic nature of humans and agree on the fundamental unity of mind and body. But, precisely because of the tangential contacts, the very growth of the humanistic movement, which has helped to popularize the role of the body in mental health, is a source of concern for many dance/movement therapists. Just as many humanists are worried about the proliferation of pseudohumanists with gimmick approaches (see Chapter 2), so

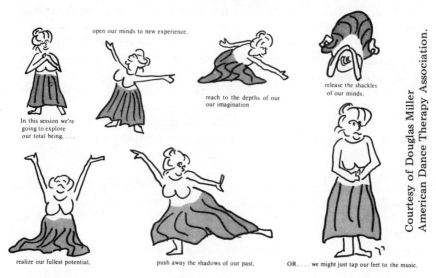

open our minds to new experience.

reach to the depths of our
our imagination

release the shackles
of our minds,

In this session we're
going to explore
our total being, . . .

realize our fullest potential,

push away the shadows of our past.

OR. . . . we might just tap our feet to the music.

Courtesy of Douglas Miller
American Dance Therapy Association.

some in dance/movement are alarmed at the collection of body movement "gimmicks" in supermarket fashion by some primarily verbal psychotherapists. Too many group "facilitators," they believe, use these techniques without understanding underlying principles of movement or fitting them into a coherent and meaningful context. Many groups that have rushed to "use" nonverbal techniques are led by individuals who have had little more training than some graduate courses in counseling at a state university, or an in-house program offered by an "institute" for several weeks or months. Few of those outside the ranks of dance/movement therapists have had more than a fleeting contact with kinesiology, movement analysis, movement notation, or principles of effort/shape.

From another direction has come the intrusion of the bandwagon riders who are associated with dance in other contexts — recreational, performing, aesthetic, or social — and who want to participate in the growing popularity of the somatic therapies. Large numbers of "slimnastics" and "dancersize" teachers have been using the words "therapy" and "therapeutic" in their advertising, and even teachers of ballroom dancing and jazz routines have been proclaiming to the world their availability to provide "dance therapy."

Trained and experienced dance/movement therapists are still relatively scarce in the mental health field. However, growing numbers each year work in psychiatric hospitals, clinics, day treatment centers, schools for exceptional children, homes for the aged, referral agencies, correctional institutions, private practice, and — more recently — research.

In recent years, some dance/movement therapists have advanced the bold assertion, heard increasingly at ADTA conferences, that it is not enough for dance therapists to struggle for acceptance in adjunctive roles. Unlike practitioners in most other therapies — verbal or nonverbal — they argue, movement therapists deal directly with one major element of the psychosomatic or somatopsychic organism; it is time, they contend, for dance and movement therapists to prepare themselves for total or primary therapy roles. The implications are that dance/movement therapists either will have to undergo ancillary training in psychotherapy or will have to develop a nosology and a language that are independent of psychology and psychiatry.

Among those who adhere to the second of these views are some who point to the interrelationship between body and mind and who contend that correcting the physical problem *alone* must inevitably influence the mental functioning. This position parallels the traditional behaviorist contention that the behavior *is* the problem, not merely a manifestation of it. Nevertheless, because few dance/ movement therapists are willing to accept the methodologies of behavior therapy, little has been written on dance/movement from a behaviorist orientation.

Whether or not dance/movement therapists ever break from the psychological models, ample evidence demonstrates that many have abandoned the medical model, preferring — like most humanist psychotherapists — to see therapy as self-growth, self-improvement, and self-actualization, rather than as treatment for disorder. In April 1978, Blanche Evan, herself a pioneer dance therapist and a contemporary of Marian Chace, sent an undated open letter to all ADTA members, angrily criticizing the organization for restricting the internship experience for registry to the treatment of hospitalized psychopaths and psychotics, to the exclusion of the treatment of (education of) the "normal neurotic," the group with which she has worked for over twenty-five years.

The glaring weakness in dance/movement is in the area of research. Most of the research on which the theoretical framework has been built has come from outside the field. And the validating research, the test of dance/movement theories and practices, is in its infancy. Few carefully designed outcome studies have been conducted and fewer yet reported, a deficiency of which leaders in the field are painfully aware. The very second issue of the new *American Journal of Dance Therapy* carried an article addressing the need for solid outcome research. Describing "research" reports in the field, psychologist Daniel Millberg of the University of Pittsburgh writes that in the typical case history

> the theoretical interpretation and the therapeutic approach are accepted as an explanation for the change [that has been noted] without verification. This type of research scenario pervades dance movement therapy research. The problems of this design are innumerable including difficulties in both internal and external validity, with the major defect being a lack of appropriate control groups. Given this model, it is no wonder the results and successes of dance movement therapy techniques have not been widely accepted.[79]

The article itself, happily, coincided with evidence that small numbers of dance and movement therapists *are*, in fact, engaged in conducting and reporting carefully controlled outcome studies; it would be more accurate to interpret such comments less as a denigration of the field than as a sign of the search for direction. This search is indicated in an editorial by Joanna G. Harris in the same issue:

We are hurrying to catch up. . . . . We are catching up with our expectations, reviewing our statements of belief and intention, and making a stand toward professional validation.

We are an "emerging profession," hurrying to achieve a clear image, establish a substantial body of knowledge, provide and maintain high standards of education and practice, and earn respect from our students and colleagues.[80]

REFERENCE NOTES

1. Wilhelm Reich, *Character Analysis* (New York: Orgone Institute Press, 1945), pp. 311, 315-16, 320-21.
2. Claire Schmais, "Dance Therapy in Perspective," in *Dance Therapy*, ed. K. C. Mason (Focus on Dance, VII) (Washington, D. C.: American Association of Health, Education and Recreation, 1974).
3. Marian Chace, *Marian Chace: Her Papers*, ed. Harris Chaiklin (Columbia, Md.: American Dance Therapy Association, 1975), p. 12.
4. Schmais, "Dance Therapy in Perspective," p. 9.
5. Charles Darwin, *The Expression of the Emotions in Man and Animals* (Chicago: University of Chicago Press, 1965), p. 32.
6. Herbert Ginsburg and Sylvia Opper, *Piaget's Theory of Intellectual Development: An Introduction* (Englewood Cliffs, N.J.: Prentice-Hall, 1966); Jerome S. Bruner, R. R. Oliver, P. H. Greenfield, et al., *Studies in Cognitive Growth* (New York: John Wiley & Sons, 1966).
7. Ginsburg and Opper, *Piaget's Theory of Intellectual Development*, pp. 75-79.
8. Quoted in William C. Schutz, "Encounter," in *Current Psychotherapies*, ed. Raymond Corsini (Itasca, Ill.: F. E. Peacock, 1973), p. 421.
9. Edmund Jacobson, *Progressive Relaxation* (Chicago: University of Chicago Press, 1938).
10. Edmund Jacobson, *Biology of Emotions* (Springfield, Ill.: Charles C Thomas, 1967).
11. Wilder Penfield and Lamar Roberts, *Speech and Brain Mechanisms* (Princeton, N.J.: Princeton University Press, 1959).
12. Ida Rolf, *Structural Integration* (New York: Viking Press, 1972).
13. Ray L. Birdwhistell, *Kinesics and Context* (Philadelphia: University of Pennsylvania Press, 1970).
14. Ibid., p. 24.
15. William S. Condon and W. D. Ogston, "Sound-Film Analysis of Normal and Pathological Behavior Patterns," *Journal of Nervous and Mental Disease* 143 (1966):338-47.
16. William S. Condon, "Linguistic-Kinesic Research and Dance Therapy," *Proceedings*, Third Annual Conference of the American Dance Therapy Association, 1968 (Baltimore: ADTA, 1969), p. 34.

17. Ibid., p. 37.
18. Lawrence Blair, *Rhythms of Vision* (New York: Warner Books, 1975).
19. William S. Condon and L. W. Sander, "Neonate Movement Is Synchronized with Adult Speech: Interactional Participation and Language Acquisition," *Science* 183 (1974):99–101.
20. Judith S. Kestenberg and Arnhilt Buelte, "Prevention, Infant Therapy and the Treatment of Adults," *International Journal of Psychoanalytic Psychotherapy* 6 (1977):347.
21. Birdwhistell, *Kinesics and Context*.
22. Kestenberg and Buelte, "Prevention, Infant Therapy and the Treatment of Adults," p. 349.
23. Sigmund Freud, "Fragment of an Analysis of a Case of Hysteria," (1905) in *Collected Works* (London: Hogarth Press, 1924), p. 94.
24. Warren Lamb, *Posture and Gesture: An Introduction to the Study of Physical Behavior* (London: Gerald Duckworth, 1965), p. 10.
25. Marion North, *Personality Assessment Through Movement* (Boston: Plays, 1972); Alexander Lowen, *The Language of the Body* (New York: Collier Books, 1958); Albert E. Scheflen, "The Significance of Posture in Communication Systems," *Psychiatry* 27 (1964):316–31.
26. Lamb, *Posture and Gesture*, p. 11.
27. Arnold Gesell, *The First Five Years of Life* (New York: Harper and Brothers, 1940).
28. Reich, *Character Analysis*.
29. F. Deutsch, "Analytic Posturology," in *Yearbook of Psychoanalysis*, ed., Lorand (New York: International Universities Press, 1953), pp. 234–49.
30. Lamb, *Posture and Gesture*.
31. Rudolf Laban and F. C. Lawrence, *Effort* (London: McDonald and Evans, 1947); Rudolf Laban and F. C. Lawrence, *Effort: Economy in Body Movement* (Boston: Plays, 1974).
32. Lamb, *Posture and Gesture*; conversations with Irmgard Bartenieff, October 1979.
33. Penny Bernstein and Enzo Cafarelli, "An Electromyographical Validation of the Effort System of Notation," in *Monograph No. 2*, American Dance Therapy Association (Columbia, Md.: ADTA, 1972), pp. 78–94.
34. Samuel Thornton, *Laban's Theory of Movement: A New Perspective* (Boston: Plays, 1971), p. 33.
35. North, *Personality Assessment Through Movement*, p. 5.
36. North, *Personality Assessment Through Movement*.
37. Taghi Modarressi, "Motor Organization and Symbolic Signification in Childhood Psychosis," *American Journal of Dance Therapy* 1 (Fall/Winter 1977):8.
38. Alexander Lowen, *The Betrayal of the Body* (Toronto, Ont.: Collier-Macmillan Canada, 1967), p. 7.
39. B. Christiansen, *Thus Speaks the Body: Attempts Toward a Personology from the Point of View of Respiration and Posture* (Oslo: Institute for Social Research, 1963; Arno reprint, 1972).

40. D. Mary Lee Trott, "Expressive Movement Style and Personality Characteristic," *Proceedings*, Ninth Annual Conference of the American Dance Therapy Association, 1974 (Columbia, Md.: ADTA, 1975), pp. 124-30.
41. Elaine V. Siegel, "Psychoanalytic Thought and Methodology in Dance/ Movement Therapy," in Mason, *Dance Therapy*, p. 28.
42. Ibid.
43. Schmais, "Dance Therapy in Perspective," p. 10.
44. Judith S. Kestenberg, personal interviews, January 21, 1977, June 8, 1977; Kestenberg and Arnhilt Buelte, *Prevention, Infant Therapy and the Treatment of Adults: Mutual Holding and Holding-Oneself-Up*, Presentation at the International Congress of Child Psychiatry, Philadelphia, 1974, reprinted in expanded form (Port Washington, N.Y.: Center for Parents and Children, n.d.).
45. Irmgard Bartenieff, "How Is the Dancing Teacher Equipped to Do Dance Therapy?" in *Monograph No. 1*, American Dance Therapy Association (Columbia, Md.: ADTA, 1971), p. 2.
46. Harris Chaiklin, "Research and the Development of a Profession," *Proceedings*, Third Annual Conference of the American Dance Therapy Association, 1968 (Baltimore, Md.: ADTA, n.d.), p. 69.
47. Bartenieff, "How Is the Dancing Teacher Equipped to Do Dance Therapy?" p. 3.
48. "The Meaning of Movement: As Human Expression and as an Artistic Communication," panel discussion, *Proceedings*, Third Annual Conference of the American Dance Therapy Association, 1968 (Baltimore, Md.: ADTA, n.d.), p. 4.
49. Personal observation, Sarasota Guidance Clinic Day Treatment Center, September 1978.
50. Miriam Salus and Rachel Schanberg, "Body Movement and Creative Expression for the Preschool Language Handicapped Child," in *Monograph No. 1*, American Dance Therapy Association (Columbia, Md.: ADTA, 1971), p. 38.
51. Virginia Dryansky, "A Case Study of a Chronic Paranoid Schizophrenic in Dance Therapy," in *Monograph No. 3*, American Dance Therapy Association (Columbia, Md.: ADTA, 1973-1974), p. 110.
52. Ernst Gellhorn, "Motion and Emotion: The Role of Proprioception in the Philosophy and Pathology of the Emotions," *Psychological Review* 71 (1964):457-72.
53. Paul Schilder, *The Image and Appearance of the Human Body* (New York: International Universities Press, 1955), pp. 207-08.
54. Lowen, *The Betrayal of the Body*, p. 8.
55. Birdwhistell, *Kinesics and Context*; Bernard Feder and Elaine Feder, "Smiles," *Human Behavior* (December 1978):43-45.
56. Condon, "Linguistic-Kinesic Research and Dance Therapy," p. 38.
57. L. Eisenberg and L. Kanner, "Early Infantile Autism," *American Journal of Orthopsychiatry* 26 (1956):556-66.
58. Miriam R. Berger, "Bodily Experience and Expression of Emotion," in *Monograph No 2*, American Dance Therapy Association, p. 221.

59. Mitchell L. Dratman, "Reorganization of Psychic Structures in Autism: A Study Using Body Movement Therapy," *Proceedings*, Second Annual Conference of the American Dance Therapy Association (Columbia, Md.: ADTA, 1971), p. 42.
60. Penny Bernstein and Lawrence Bernstein, "A Conceptualization of Group Dance-Movement Therapy as a Ritual Process," in *Monograph No. 3*, ADTA, p. 121.
61. Trudi Schoop with Peggy Mitchell, *Won't You Join the Dance: A Dancer's Essay Into the Treatment of Psychosis* (Palo Alto, Calif.: National Press Books, 1974), pp. 146–47.
62. Quoted in Jesse D. Geller, "Dance Therapy as Viewed by a Psychotherapist," in *Monograph No. 3*, ADTA, p. 4.
63. Reuben Fine, "Psychoanalysis," in *Current Psychotherapies*, ed. Raymond Corsini, p. 21.
64. Schoop, *Won't You Join the Dance*, p. 146.
65. Ibid.
66. John Heider, "Catharsis in Human Potential Encounter," *Journal of Humanistic Psychology* 14, no. 4 (Fall 1974):32.
67. Beth Kalish, "Body Movement Therapy for Autistic Children," *Proceedings*, Third Annual Conference, ADTA, p. 51.
68. S. Tarachow, *An Introduction to Psychotherapy* (New York: International Universities Press, 1963), p. 96.
69. Albert E. Scheflen with Alice Scheflen, *Body Language and Social Order* (Englewood Cliffs, N.J.: Prentice-Hall, 1972); Albert E. Scheflen, "Quasi-Courtship Behavior in Psychotherapy," *Psychiatry* 28 (1965):245–57.
70. Schoop, *Won't You Join the Dance*, p. 149.
71. Ibid., pp. 149–50.
72. Scheflen, *Body Language and Social Order*, p. xiii.
73. S. Schachter, "The Interaction of Cognitive and Physiological Determinants of Emotional State," in *Advances in Experimental Social Psychology*, ed. L. Berkowitz (New York: Academic Press, 1964).
74. Benjamin Wolman, ed., *The Therapist's Handbook* (New York: Van Nostrand Reinhold, 1976), p. 307.
75. Chace, *Marian Chace: Her Papers*; Elaine V. Siegel, "The Resolution of Breast Fixations in Three Schizophrenic Teenagers During Movement Therapy," *Proceedings*, Fifth Annual Conference of the American Dance Therapy Association, 1970 (Columbia, Md.: ADTA, 1971), pp. 59–70.
76. Mary Whitehouse, "The Transference and Dance Therapy," *American Journal of Dance Therapy* 1, no. 1 (Spring/Summer 1977):4.
77. Janet A. Boettinger, "Integrity of Body and Psyche: Some Notes on Work in Process," *Proceedings*, Seventh Annual Conference of the American Dance Therapy Association, 1972 (Kensington, Md.: ADTA, 1973), p. 48.
78. Schmais, "Dance Therapy in Perspective," p. 9.
79. Daniel B. Millberg, "Directions for Research in Dance Movement Therapy," *American Journal of Dance Therapy* 1, no. 2 (Fall/Winter 1977):16.
80. Joanne G. Harris, "Editor's Effort: Writing About Dance Therapy," *American Journal of Dance Therapy* 1, no. 2 (Fall/Winter 1977):2.

EFFORT/SHAPE MOVEMENT
ANALYSIS

Rudolf Laban has probably done more than any other individual to systematize the analysis and notation of movement. His basic notation system, called *kinetography* in Europe and *Labanotation* in the United States, is widely used to describe direction, body part, weight transference, and duration of movement. Since its introduction in 1928, it has become a standard method of dance notation.

Of more interest to dance/movement therapists is Laban's work in the qualitative analysis of movement, in terms of *how* movement is performed and how *effort* can be analyzed in terms of its components: space, weight, time, and flow. The system has been modified by a number of others, particularly Warren Lamb and Marion North, English disciples of Laban, and Irmgard Bartenieff, who was instrumental in introducing the system in this country.

The system is based on a simple grid that Laban used to describe effort. Laban thought of weight as light or strong, and flow (or control) as free or bound.

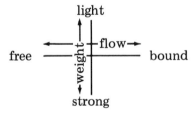

An accent sign, denoting effort, is central to the notation system.

This sign of effort separates the components for notation purposes.

Weight

light

Flow ——— free / bound

strong

Individual notations would indicate

Flow free   bound

Weight light   strong

The element of *time* is indicated by notations for *sustained* movement or *sudden* movement and is shown on the basic grid by the addition of a horizontal line parallel to the *flow* line.

Time indications

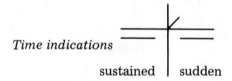

sustained | sudden

The element of *space* is indicated on the basic grid by lines added to the upper right quadrant.

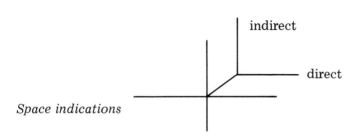

Space indications

The total grid, indicating weight, flow, time, and space, appears as follows.

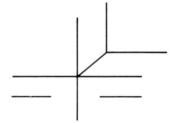

In application, the components of the grid can be isolated for the notation of movement from a classical ballet to an industrial worker's physical variations at his work.

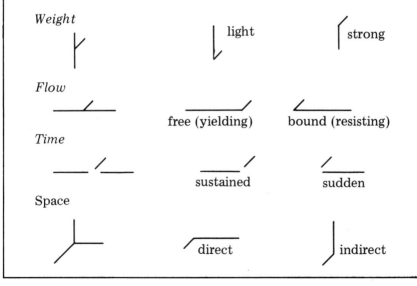

Warren Lamb contributed to the grid the component of *shape* by simply adding an additional diagonal.

Separated from the basic grid, the symbols for *shape flow* and *shape qualities* appear as follows:

Flow of Shape: movement that goes toward or away from the body.

growing or unfolding (scattering)

shrinking or folding (gathering)

Qualities of Shape: movement that relates to the outside world.

Horizontal

widening

narrowing

Vertical

rising

sinking

Sagittal

advancing

retreating

The *Dance Notation Bureau* (505 Eighth Avenue, New York, N.Y. 10018) and the *Laban Institute of Movement Studies* (133 West 21st Street, New York, N.Y. 10011) offer workshops, courses, and certification programs in *Labanotation*, *Effort/Shape Movement Analysis*, and related movement analysis and notation systems.

Detailed descriptions of movement analysis and notation may be found in Marion North, *Personality Assessment Through Movement* (London: Macdonald and Evans, 1972; New York: Plays, 1975); Valerie Preston-Dunlop, *A Handbook for Modern Educational Dance* (London: Macdonald and Evans, 1963); and Cecily Dell, *A Primer for Movement Description Using Effort-Shape and Supplementary Concepts* (New York: Dance Notation Bureau, 1970). A recent work is *Body Movement: Coping with the Environment*, by Irmgard Bartenieff, founder of the *Laban Institute of Movement Studies*, in collaboration with Dori Lewis (New York: Gordon and Breach, Science Publishers, 1980).

FOLK DANCE
IN DANCE THERAPY

In the day treatment or day care centers that have developed in many community mental health programs, the care of patients is quite different from that in mental hospitals. The major goal of many such centers is to "contain" their populations — to keep patients out of hospitals. In some programs, an attempt is also made to reintegrate patients into the work force. The quality and scope of treatment varies widely among centers; for the most part, the services provided are quite limited, and individual "deep" therapy is rarely undertaken. While there is often a core of "regulars," the patient populations usually include numbers of transients. Programs, therefore, tend to focus on short-term objectives, many of them "objectives of opportunity" that arise out of specific problems or situations.

The use of folk dance may be a particularly useful device in such settings as a nonthreatening form of therapeutic movement or as an introduction to other forms of dance/movement therapy. In a day treatment center, the following may be the more-or-less fixed goals of the dance therapy program:

1. To expand the movement range and vocabulary of the patients by using varied rhythms and movement styles, and to help structure the often amorphous or inchoate movements of the individuals. Within the structure, a good deal of opportunity can be provided for self-expression.
2. To promote body awareness, as the patients see themselves and their movements in relation to others.
3. To provide "coping" mechanisms by teaching patients to identify and correct body distortions, and to relieve their physical tensions (and, presumably, their mental counterparts).
4. To encourage socialization through group activities in which individuals acquire a sense of belonging to a group, sharpen their abilities to interpret accurately the "body language" of others, and have an opportunity to

test their own communication systems in a free and encouraging group atmosphere.

Folk dances provide stereotyped and stylized patterns that are often acceptable to patients who might resist spontaneous movement. Moreover, the rhythms themselves are often energizing and inviting. Patients often (and quite erroneously) assume that such patterned movements are not revealing or self-disclosing.

The number of possible variations in movement patterns, styles of stance and movement, and rhythms is so great that the therapist who is knowledgeable in folk dance can quickly draw from a repertory of dances to achieve a variety of specific objectives. For example:

To promote socialization. Any of the many circle dances, such as the *kolos*, *oros*, and *drmses* of Yugoslavia, immediately help to establish group cohesion. In addition, a circle formation permits participants to join or leave a group at will. The "mixers" that can be found among the folk dances of most nationalities provide for casual interaction with a number of individuals. The therapist who thinks that the opportunity is appropriate to encourage proximity may choose one of the many Turkish line dances that call for close shoulder-to-shoulder positioning. The Greek *miteritsa* forces a quick choice of a new partner — of the opposite sex — and may be used for encouraging both decision making and the acceptance of one's sexuality.

To encourage large, free movements. Marian Chace found that waltzes have an almost universal appeal and that they encourage free movement — and conversation. At St. Elizabeth's Hospital, she remarked on a number of occasions, all sessions began with waltz music. Waltz rhythms can be used for "free movement" or for led dances, and both stimulate large whole body movement. Waltz dances can be used, in addition, for ancillary purposes. The *family waltz*, for example, can be used to explore the concept of "passing" — and controlling — a partner. Such whole body movements are encouraged in a number of nationality dances, including many of the Italian *tarantellas*.

To explore nonverbal communication. Investigating the phenomenon of interactional synchrony, William S. Condon remarked that moving together in harmony *is* communication (see Chapter 5). But each nationality or ethnic group expresses in its folk dance a stance and movement "accent." Hungarian dances, for example, stress pride and bearing; Spanish and Italian dances exhibit sexual exuberance; Ukrainian peasant dances put a premium on exhibitionism and the freedom to extemporize; some, like the subtle *cherechna* of Macedonia focus on sensitivity and adjustment to the rhythms and movements of others in the group. Virtually every nationality has dances that incorporate stereotyped "qualifiers" that make it clear that apparently sexually suggestive or aggressive movements are not to be taken literally. The gradual acceptance of such gestural qualifiers adds to the ability to interpret accurately the specifics of nonverbal communication.

To experiment with leading and following. Such dances as the Macedonian *savila se bela losa* or the Peruvian *carnevalita* are "two-headed"; a leader at each end takes over as the rhythm changes and leads the line at his or her discretion. Many Greek line dances involve the passing of leadership to others in the line.

To explore timing and rhythm. Not only are the rhythm qualities of different nationality dances themselves sufficiently different to provide variations, but many incorporate dramatic rhythmic and movement changes within the same dance. The Serbian *ersko kolo* is a circle dance that is useful when there is a disproportionate number of men and women; the Mexican *la raspa* is a couple's dance that includes rhythm changes, and the Polish *troyak* is a triad, as the name suggests. The Rumanian *ciuleandra*, unlike these rhythmic contrast dances, provides for a progressive acceleration of a basic rhythm and movement pattern.

To relieve tensions and aggressions. Many Rumanian dances, in particular, and some German dances, call for a good deal of vigorous foot stamping — the louder the better.

To explore variations in the flow of effort and shape. Some dances, like the Japanese *tonko bushi*, provide a wide range of possibilities in the application of effort and shape flow; they can be performed in a variety of ways, and they may help patients to recognize the possibility of alternatives and options within a structure.

To encourage humor and enjoyment. Good humor, and particularly shared humor, is therapeutic in itself; it is an aspect of a healthy personality. Some dances, like the Czech *doudlebska polka*, the Scandinavian *ox tanz*, and the German *hammarschmiedgeselln*, evoke laughter — even if the dancers are not completely successful in their endeavors.

What distinguishes the use of folk dance in therapy from folk dance as recreation is purpose. The focus in therapy is not on proficiency or dance style, or on the perfection of ethnic quality. It may be on the basic structure of movement, or it may be the evocation of mood, or it may be on shared experience. The therapist must be more sensitive than the folk dance teacher to the needs of the group at the moment and so chooses the dances for therapeutic purposes. She will pick up the prevailing mood or rhythm of the group at the beginning of a session, and only gradually will she introduce change — and then for a therapeutic purpose.

The mastery of dance style or the specifics of foot patterns are not at the heart of the activity; the freedom to deviate or to improvise is integral to the use of dance in therapy. As Marian Chace put it, patients need to be able to test whether they are still free to act as they wish within a group; it is the task of the dance therapy leader "to permit enough freedom to exist for the patients to move with individual, personal responses, yet remain a cohesive group." (Harris Chaiklin, ed., *Marian Chace: Her Papers* [Columbia, Md.: American Dance Therapy Association, 1975], pp. 76, 155.) However, the way patients perform movements may provide feedback to the therapist — and to themselves — on their ability to coordinate and "get it all together."

The therapist must be aware that the folk dances are devices to be used for specific purposes, and should be considered neither the totality of a dance therapy program, nor, if they are to be considered therapy, mere recreational activities. Problems may arise that call for additional movement work — exercises in relaxation, for example, or breathing, or centering. Feelings may be aroused that call for discussion, in the group or later during psychotherapy. Individual movement patterns may disclose problems that will require follow-up. Folk dancing is not dance therapy, but it can be a useful technique in dance therapy.

Adapted from a book in preparation by Elaine Feder on the use of group movement in community mental health programs and in special education.

AARON JOINS THE WORLD

Mrs. W began to feel concern for her son Aaron as he approached his first birthday. His motor development seemed normal, but she wondered why he did not respond to her and was always busy spinning objects. As he grew older, it became increasingly apparent that Aaron was slow in speech development and in toilet training. He avoided contact with his father and his two older brothers, and his contact with his mother seemed limited to situations in which he wanted something done for him. In addition, he was hyperactive and threw temper tantrums.

A month before Aaron's second birthday, Mrs. W saw a television program about autistic children — children who seem unable or unwilling to form human relationships and who seem to withdraw into a private world. Mrs. W began to suspect that Aaron was autistic. After a number of clinical examinations, Aaron was, in fact, diagnosed as autistic and was then referred to the Developmental Center for Autistic Children in Philadelphia. He was admitted to the center in September 1970, shortly before his third birthday.

Aaron exhibited many symptoms of autism: withdrawal from personal relationships, repetition of stereotyped movements, a failure to develop communicative language, an inability to imitate, fascination with small inanimate objects. However, some of his behavior was not typical of autistic behavior; for example, he was alert to his surroundings, could differentiate between people, and could, when adequately motivated, master simple tasks that he would perform with apparent enjoyment. The members of the clinical team — psychoanalyst, psychologist, special teacher, speech therapist, movement therapist, and social worker — concluded that Aaron "presents mixed symptomology of a child with ego disturbance resulting from a possible minimal brain damage with secondary autism."

A major characteristic of minimally brain damaged children is a distorted or undeveloped sense of body image, an inability to discern accurately where their body boundaries end and the outside world begins. A distorted body image must inevitably affect a child's self-concept. However, children with minimal brain damage are amenable to treatment, and the prognosis for change is excellent. Body movement therapy, therefore, was seen as an integral part of Aaron's treatment plan.

During the first two weeks Aaron was in the center, he was given an opportunity to adjust to the new surroundings, with his mother, and sometimes his father, present. The staff observed family interaction, and body movement therapist Beth Kalish notated the movement patterns of both parents in order to learn something about the nonverbal messages Aaron might be receiving from them. Among her findings: Mr. W moved with "staccato-like spurts of energy" when he interacted with Aaron. "He will pick him up jerkily from behind and toss him gleefully into the air. Aaron's movements freeze and become bound, as he looks on the verge of a panic response."

In the early movement therapy sessions, Aaron's movement behavior and speech patterns were hyperactive and erratic. He would often seem to be in the middle of a tantrum when he would stop to point to an object, such as a light bulb, say "light," and look at Dr. Kalish as though for an answer. The speech therapist suggested that any such verbalization should be accepted and answered in a complete sentence. By incorporating the word in a more meaningful context, those who worked with Aaron might help him to break through the labeling and pointing behaviors through which Aaron and the other members of his family had communicated. Kalish found that this technique also gave Aaron "a way out of his so-called tantrum behavior."

The movement therapy sessions focused on movement interaction designed to help Aaron build a more realistic body image. Kalish joined Aaron in jumping over a balance board, climbing on steps, and running in front of a large mirror, in which Aaron could see both himself and the therapist. Increasingly, Aaron began to imitate the movements of the therapist. "We were recreating the mother-infant learning model," she reports. In time, more and more of each session began to involve physical contact, although Aaron still resisted such contact. His eye contact "improved from intermittent glances to long steady looks when our faces were on the same level." After a number of sessions, Kalish reported that "now there was meaningful interaction. We would roll on the floor together or run to the mirror until tired." After six weeks of therapy sessions, the temper tantrums were gone; there was a more directed and purposeful approach to other activities outside the therapy sessions.

Because Aaron was out sick for a few days, his schedule was disrupted. The next time Kalish went to get him for movement therapy, he was in the playroom with his mother. When he saw the therapist, Aaron had a temper tantrum, and the mother was reluctant to let him go. As soon as Aaron and Kalish were in the therapy room with the door closed, the screaming stopped abruptly. To Kalish, the tantrum was a way of testing both mother and therapist. The mother's response, she thought, was ambivalent. Mrs. W was as fearful of separation as was Aaron, and she sent him a message of distrust of the therapist; at the same time, she was probably expressing anger at the fact that the therapist was able to cope with Aaron better than she.

For such reasons, the mothers of the children at the center were involved in a (verbal) psychotherapy group and in a movement therapy group that Kalish had instituted "for relaxation." The therapist's purpose, in Mrs. W's case, was to help the mother to develop a more positive self-concept and to release her own tensions. The achievement of such goals would, in the long run, help Aaron as much as Mrs. W. After a number of weeks, reported the therapist, "Mrs. W is now more relaxed in body attitude. . . . Her interaction with other group members has increased, her posture is more alert and there is less tension around the mouth, face and shoulders."

For Aaron, there were even stronger indications of progress. Because he was essentially a nonverbal child, "observational," rather than verbal tests were used to measure his progress. Kalish used the *Behavior Rating Instrument for Autistic and Other Atypical Children* (BRIAAC) during the third and ninth weeks. This test, developed by Kalish, B. Ruttenberg, C. Wenar, and E. Wolf, and published by Stoelting and Co. (1350 S. Kostner Avenue, Chicago, Ill., 60623) measures developmental levels in eight areas: relationship, communication, vocalization, speech and sound reception, social functioning, body movement, psychosexual development, and drive for mastery. Aaron showed marked improvement in the areas of relationships, communication, and movement. The relationship score, reads the report, "indicates a solid base on which the Child Care Worker can now begin to work to improve Aaron's score on the mastery scale," an area that had not been stressed up to that time. By the time of the second test, Aaron no longer needed medication for hyperactivity. Kalish's report concludes:

> As he improves in the areas of speech and communication skills, he will be ready to move from the present placement into a small group of developmentally delayed children with a sensitive teacher who can help him learn to relate to his peers. He will need experiences with children his own age before he will be ready to move into a normal school setting. If he continues to improve at the present rate, his prognosis of reaching his age level is encouraging.

Shortly before the publication of this book, Kalish wrote to say: "When I last heard, Aaron had continued to progress, as predicted, and was in an age-appropriate class with normal children."

Adapted from an unpublished case report by Beth Kalish, Ph.D., D.T.R., Director of Movement Therapy Graduate Program, Loyola Marymount University, Los Angeles, California. Dr. Kalish is a past president of ADTA.

"THAT WAS A TRIP"

Dance therapist Liljan Espenak had been intrigued for some time with the concepts underlying ritual "shamanistic" dances that induced trance states and ecstasy. In particular, she thought, the trances that accompanied the twirling of the whirling dervishes seemed to conform with some recent thinking in dance therapy theory. The monotonous turns themselves might permit, in her words, "an inward gaze and contemplation . . . a realization of center, a real discovery of strength and power." Could not such trance states serve as a bridge over which some of her clients could escape their reliance on drugs for "highs"?

C, a young girl from a well-to-do family, found herself isolated from others, bored, and "uptight." She had dropped out of school and had turned to sex and drugs. Espenak's early work with C involved a movement assessment. C's rigid back and the general tension in her joints suggested to the therapist a reflection of an emotional rigidity. "Her back was 'proud,'" reported Espenak. "She was not going to give in to anything or anybody." C said that she liked to dance. When she was asked to improvise, she chose a rock record and began to move mechanically. "Her pelvis was practically immobile, with the movement mainly in the knees and twisting shoulders," noted the therapist, who inferred that C's "frozen rigidity" in movement was symptomatic of an absence of feeling or meaning in other areas of her life.

The first movement sessions, involving relaxation and breathing, met with a good deal of resistance from C, who apparently fought the idea of freeing her body from control. Espenak's assessment involved a conversion of movement qualities into character traits. She assessed C as very high in dynamic drive, courage, endurance, and self-assurance (or ego image). Her weakness in physical coordination, on the other hand, suggested "low emotional state" and "control of drive."

Espenak decided to make use of the whirling movements of the dervishes as a way of forcing C to relinquish ego control of her body. C was given exercises to help her in "coordination in progression." When she began to perform the actual whirls, her legs turned, while her torso and arms resisted; C became violently nauseated, a reaction that the therapist interpreted, in part, as "a psychosomatic method of getting out of the uncomfortable demands made upon her courage."

The turns were modified so that the direction would change after every eight counts; the seven steps in each sequence could involve one, two, or three rotations, so that C could make a conscious choice of tempo and degree of turn. Session after session saw C turning, striving to make the turns mechanically better. One day, as the turning began, C began to twirl without changing direction and without stopping. "She turned and turned," said Espenak, "faster and faster, almost as in anger, certainly in ecstasy," until she fell on the floor, where she rolled a few times before coming to a stop. The therapist watched in silence. After a while, C spoke. "That was a trip," she said.

Adapted from Liljan Espenak, D.T.R., "Trance and Ecstasy in Dance Therapy," in ADTA, *Proceedings*, Ninth Annual Conference, 1974, pp. 103–17. By permission of Liljan Espenak and the ADTA. Espenak is an assistant professor at the New York Medical College, and teaches postgraduate dance therapy at Flower Hospital in New York City. She is a dance therapist at the Alfred Adler Mental Health Clinic, and the author of *Dance Therapy: Theory and Application*, Springfield, Illinois: Charles C Thomas, 1981.

MOVEMENT AND A
DEPRESSED NEUROTIC

L was an unmarried woman who lived alone. She had been referred to movement therapist Dianne Dulicai by a psychiatrist who had diagnosed L as suffering from neurotic depression. He thought that intervention at the body movement level would be more effective than verbal therapy. When L appeared at the first movement therapy session, she complained of a feeling of "lifelessness" and said that she was "disconnected from any feelings" and had no desires to do anything.

In her assessment, Dulicai recorded L's movements and interpreted the pattern as "displaying predominance of passive weight and even fluctuations of free to bound flow." (In her case summary, Dulicai adds, "In non-technical language, she looked like a limp dishrag consoling itself by rocking.") L's upper body was sunken and retreated, her pelvis inactive, her head lowered, apparently to avoid eye contact. Her movements were weak, unclear, and indecisive.

Dulicai was less interested in the possible psychoanalytic diagnosis (perhaps midlife reactive depression with oral rhythms) or behavioral interpretation (inappropriate coping mechanism) than in her own movement assessment. To Dulicai, movement therapy can operate effectively for many problems without a theoretical base from any other therapy or discipline. If the psyche and the soma are interdependent and continually inter-acting aspects of the individual, then it is just as effective to deal directly with the soma first as it would be for a verbal therapist to begin with the verbal aspects of the psyche. Changes in physical stance and in movement patterns must inevitably influence psychic aspects of the individual.

Focusing on body movement change, Dulicai concluded that "the treatment of choice for me is to use the movement data and build on untapped physical resources. Whatever the psychological influences or my interpretation of the causes of the movement problems, the movement data are sufficient as a base from which to make change." Dulicai's thinking was that L's restricted movements were a manifestation of her depression; by expanding her range of movements ("expansion of possibilities"), L's behavior itself would change. Her choices would be based on a wider range of options; moreover, she would be more likely than before to make independent and autonomous decisions.

Dulicai worked on L's body alignment, which involved, among other things, freeing and activating the pelvic area. L's posture was improved, permitting her to breathe more deeply ("to take what she needs to survive," writes Dulicai), but also raising for discussion L's self-consciousness about being flat-chested. The course of movement therapy sessions inevitably raised issues of eye contact and interpersonal relationships.

Looking back at the case of L, Dulicai notes that L "has improved her job status, has not reported feeling depressed in the last eight months, and has begun an intimate relationship with which she is struggling." On the basis of her knowledge of L, Dulicai is reasonably sure that the expansion of L's movement range has played a large role in influencing the changes that have taken place.

Adapted from case notes by Dianne Dulicai, M.A., D.T.R., Assistant Professor and Director of Dance Therapy Education, Hahnemann Medical College, Philadelphia, Pennsylvania.

SYMBIOSIS

Mary was brought to the Sheppard Pratt Hospital in Maryland after her family had prevented her from jumping out of a second-story window. For about a year, since she had left college, Mary had been showing increasing signs of mental disturbance and had been in psychotherapy. Shortly before the suicide attempt, she had been having hallucinations, was urinating on the beds of other family members, and was screaming that she was possessed by the devil. At the hospital, she was described as scared, suspicious, disorganized, with loose associations and delusions. She had difficulty speaking in sentences; much of the time, she had hallucinations; and she believed that she was possessed by demons. At times, she would be quite catatonic and mute. A few weeks after her admission to the hospital, Mary tried to set fire to her room.

At the time dance therapist Arlynne Stark began to work with her, Mary had become quite a problem for staff and for fellow patients. She was unable to take care of even her simplest needs; she was too disorganized and confused to dress herself, to brush her teeth or to bathe, and required almost continuous attention. Stark reports:

> After conferring with members of the treatment team I began to formulate some specific goals for our work together. First, I wanted to establish a relationship through nonverbal communication so that she could begin to define a sense of herself and a feeling of body integration, then allow her to have the opportunity to experience and express and thereby differentiate her confused and disorganized states, affects, and thoughts in a supportive situation. By exploring these in movement I wanted to move the material from the unconscious and preverbal into consciousness and verbal material so that she could begin to integrate the interrelationship between her affect, thoughts and behaviors.

Stark saw her role as that of a "catalyst." She began by mirroring and reflecting back with her own body the expressions of Mary's movements. "I became a screen for her to view herself," Stark writes, "so that she would begin to gain a sense of her own self and a sense of her own experience." It was almost impossible for Mary to follow verbal directions or to follow the therapist's movements, so Stark responded to Mary's own movements and feelings. "Nonverbally I was trying to tell her that I could accept her at the level at which she was functioning. . . . By first picking up, mirroring, and then enlarging and developing or expanding what I observed in movement, movement dialogues and themes began to emerge. As with all my work as a dance therapist, verbal material was used to reinforce the awareness of experience." While individual sessions were not focused on predetermined specific objectives, themes did emerge out of the movement patterns.

From the very beginning, the dance therapy dealt with helping Mary to define herself through body awareness and "body boundary" work, so that she could distinguish between the world within and the world outside her own body.

During the first session, Stark picked up from Mary's movements the theme of approach and avoidance. Mary vacillated between approaching the therapist and moving away from her. Stark and Mary spent a good deal of that session walking around the room. When Mary approached Stark, the therapist responded with similar movements, which almost always would provoke a tensing up and a backing away; Stark's response here, too, was a reflection, this time of avoidance. At times, they simply walked around the room together, with Stark accommodating herself to Mary's rhythm and movements, at times varying her style so that Mary could sense the difference between them.

Like most severely disturbed patients, Mary did not have a clearly defined body image. During some of the early dance therapy sessions, Mary and the therapist began to approach each other with hands outstretched. But when they made contact, Mary's fingers continued to move toward the therapist. "It felt as though she was going to continue moving her fingers through mine," reports Stark, who responded with a gentle pressure in order to help Mary recognize her own body boundaries and those of the therapist. After a few weeks, Mary was better able to recognize where she ended and the therapist began. On occasion, her confusion still showed. She would put on the therapist's shoes and claim that she was Arlynne

Stark; from time to time, she would call the therapist "Mary."

For a time, they worked in front of a mirror to provide Mary with visual as well as tactile feedback. "Still she touched my arm and claimed it was hers," Stark says. "At times, I moved away from her and the mirror so she would be able to see only her own reflection."

Stark saw mirroring as a way of reflecting not only body boundaries and movement, but expression as well. She says:

> By using my body the same way she is using hers, and paying particular attention to the expressive components, I am able to provide a mirror, an objective view of what she is doing. In this way she begins to acquire a recognition of what she might be feeling.
>
> Mary and I stand facing each other about four feet apart. I am moving with her, our movements synchronous. As she begins to curl her fingers into tight clenched fists, I follow with the same gesture. Her body tenses slightly as she holds her clenched fists away from her body. I, too, tighten, and I exaggerate slightly the "holding-on-to-clenched-fists" posture. I attempt to reflect back to her the angry tone of her movements. Looking at me, she begins to pound her fists in the air.

After Stark and Mary had been working together for some time, "we were definitely into symbiosis." Mary looked constantly at the therapist, followed her around, imitated her movements, and attempted to maintain eye contact with her for as long as possible. At times, she refused to leave when the session was over and had to be dragged out of the room by nursing staff. "She clung to the door, the wall, or me," Stark says. "Once she refused to leave and compromised by leaving her shoes. I felt this was a symbolic statement of her wanting to continue to be part of my life. . . . It was time to begin working on separation and differentiation." In one session

> we walked around the room. Mary stayed very close to my side, never taking her eyes away from me. I suggested that we hold hands and walk and look straight ahead to where we were going. By suggesting this physical contact through holding hands I had wanted to provide her with the security that I was there with her even if she could not see me. When she became comfortable with this, I suggested we let go and walk side by side, looking straight ahead. . . . I wanted her to trust the internalized memory and recognition

of my existence. . . . Eventually we worked up to moving around the room and staying far apart from each other while not looking at each other.

Mary eventually was able to tolerate longer periods of independence. She and the therapist took turns "performing" for each other, a technique by which Stark attempted to encourage Mary to move by herself.

The outcome reveals the degree to which a therapist may become personally involved in a case. Some considerable time after the events described above, Stark brought herself to write:

As Mary began to improve, she had some difficulty confronting the issues of individuation and responsibility of self. The staff and I gradually increased our expectations for appropriate behavior. Perhaps in a response to "growing up" or as an attention seeking mechanism, Mary ran away from the hospital. She returned about two weeks later and then ran away again. We heard from her family that they decided to admit her to a different hospital as Mary did not like SEPH. What is important about the ending is that the family continued to give in to her requests and did not support her treatment. [Stark had remarked in her original case report that "the family often gave in to Mary's controlling and demanding behavior."] . . . What I personally experienced as a result of the sudden interruption to our work was a feeling of loss. Because of the intensity of our work, of my own emotional investment, and the symbiosis which we shared, I felt incomplete, angry at her, and sad.

Adapted and condensed from a case history in preparation for publication by Arlynne Stark, M.A., D.T.R., and from the videotape recorded by Professor Stark, who is Director of the Dance-Movement Therapy Graduate Program, Goucher College, Towson, Maryland, and dance therapist for the Sinai Hospital Psychiatric Unit. Stark has been an officer and a member of the board of Directors of the ADTA for many years.

6

The Expressive Arts Therapies— Today and Tomorrow

Ours has been called the Age of Anxiety, the Age of Unease, and the Age of Neurosis. The implication is that our age is characterized by anxiety to a greater extent than in the past. This interpretation is possible, but what is at least as likely is that we have become increasingly self-conscious about our anxieties, our stresses, and our depressions. Moreover, we have experienced a revolution of rising expectations in mental health. Good health is no longer viewed as the absence of disease; to many, it is equated with happiness.

We have become impatient even with minor aches and pains (our time has also been called the Aspirin Age) and with the normal stresses that occur in daily living. We demand, if not necessarily cures for unhappiness, at least relief.

The increased self-consciousness and the revolution of rising expectations in mental health does not mean that the incidence of insanity has increased in modern times. Only a relatively small proportion of humanity will be stricken by madness. But increasing numbers of men and women in modern society have come to demand alleviation of their fears and their anxieties. We must differentiate here between the mental *illness* of the insane and the mental *distress* of the "normal" neurotic.

Schizophrenia, the major category of insanity, is a term that describes a variety of diseases involving brain dysfunction. Symptoms include abnormalities in *perception* (such as hearing voices or smelling odors that are not apparent to others), in *emotion* (crying or laughing inappropriately or without apparent cause), or in *thinking* (having delusions or making loose and illogical associations). These symptoms may appear once in an individual's lifetime, or they may recur, or they may be continuous. Disagreement exists, however, over whether the one-time "reactive" schizophrenia that follows a traumatic experience — and that fades with time — is true schizophrenia.

Schizophrenics the world over display the same symptoms, and every society recognizes the symptoms as those of madness. Moreover, there is general agreement that the mad suffer from a disease. The behavioral symptoms are accompanied by anatomical and biological abnormalities which, in some cases, can be controlled (not cured) through the use of drugs. The debate continues over whether the causes of schizophrenia are environmental or biological.

The traditional psychoanalytic view is that schizophrenia develops in a distorted family situation. No child is *born* with problems, according to this view; schizophrenia can be traced to damage to the child during the formative years, perhaps through some parental neglect or failure. Dr. Silvano Arieti, clinical professor of psychiatry at the New York Medical College, sees the roots of schizophrenia in a family setting that has denied the individual security or trust.[1]

In contrast, research scientists have accumulated considerable evidence that suggests a biological cause. E. Fuller Torrey, a maverick psychiatrist who has gained a reputation for breaking Freudian icons, points to the geographical distribution of schizophrenia and the strange "outbreaks" of schizophrenia in areas that had not previously known the disease, as well as to the seasonal nature of schizophrenic births. He writes: "The data appear to provide no support for psychoanalytic theories of schizophrenia (which say, for example, that it is caused by bad mothering), and little support for sociocultural theories, which hold that it is caused by cultural stress."[2]

Schizophrenics manifest clear organic and biochemical symptoms. To many, the evidence is compelling for a biological cause. "Speed freaks," using amphetamines for long periods of time, exhibit schizophrenic symptoms. Moreover, the amphetamines release dopamine, a brain neurotransmitter — a chemical messenger — that figures in several major theories of schizophrenia. One recent finding is that, while schizophrenics do not have excessive amounts of dopamine as had previously been suspected, they do have about twice the normal number of receptors for dopamine in the three areas of the brain that control emotion and motor activity.[3] The actual cause of schizophrenia is still uncertain.

In addition to the psychoanalytic contention that it is born in the bosom of the family, hypotheses of causes include environmental toxins, viruses with long latency periods (the *herpes simplex* virus, for example, produces schizophreniclike symptoms under certain conditions), and nutritional deficiencies. In any event, the standard treatment for schizophrenia today is chemotherapy, which, while it does not cure the illness, does control its symptoms. Psychotherapy has largely been abandoned as a primary treatment for schizophrenia, although it is often used with patients who are treated with drugs, in an attempt to help them cope with problems and find directions.

Like schizophrenia, the psychotic affective disorders — mania, psychotic depression, and manic-depression — are illnesses that are marked by biological symptoms. Psychotic depression is very different from "reactive" or neurotic depressions to which essentially normal and healthy individuals succumb as a result of life stresses or crises. In fact, Arieti prefers to call reactive depression "sadness."[4] In contrast with "neurotic" depression which is caused by a clearly definable situation or event — a divorce, a death, the loss of a job — psychotic depression is pervasive and undifferentiated; the individual suffering from it cannot identify the cause of the depression and is not even aware of the inappropriate nature of the emotion. As with schizophrenia, many researchers have begun to suspect a biological rather than a psychological cause. Some have amassed evidence to support a genetic cause for at least some types of manic depression.[5]

Some researchers have concluded that depression is caused by biochemical abnormalities that involve the neurotransmitters — the biogenic amines that act as messengers in the brain's transmission system—that are already suspects as causes of schizophrenia.[6] And again, as in the case of schizophrenia, the symptoms can be controlled chemically by a class of mood drugs called the tricyclic antidepressants, which are best known by such trade names as *Tofranil* and *Elavil.* According to Dr. Joseph Schildkraut of Harvard Medical School, psychotherapy and placebos are both inadequate in treating depression, for which only psychopharmacology promises effective control.[7]

While the biological basis for depression seems to be gaining adherents, there are those who cling to the traditional Freudian theory. Says Arieti: "In my opinion, there is always a psychological reason. . . . Now, I am not able to deny that certain people are biologically predisposed to be depressed, whereas others are not. But in most cases, the patient has . . . a psychological force . . . that almost ineluctably will lead him or her to depression."[8] Because, to Arieti, the cause of psychotic depression is psychological, the cure must be through psychotherapy. The fact that certain drugs help control the symptoms of depression, he argues, "doesn't mean very much because we know that many drugs are able to alter the proper functions of the nervous system."[9] Not only the powerful antidepressants, he says, but even tranquilizers and alcohol can alter moods but will not change the circumstances or touch the underlying problem.

This distinction, however, has had little practical influence on the treatment of psychotics. Overwhelmingly, the primary treatment for psychotics is psychopharmacological, because the patient in many cases is unreachable with psychotherapy unless the symptoms are controlled. If psychotherapy is used, it tends to be employed for adjunctive purposes by most psychiatrists—to help the patient cope with personal problems.

The use of art therapy and dance/movement therapy in the treatment of psychotic patients has been concentrated largely in the diagnostic function. It is widely speculated that the arts therapies can be effective in the therapeutic functions, where they can provide nonverbal experiences for patients who may have difficulty verbalizing their feelings or their thinking. Case studies suggest that dance/movement therapy may help patients recognize the conflicts between the realities of the world, as experienced through their bodies, and the delusions that color their thinking. Describing the case history of a patient diagnosed as a paranoid schizophrenic, dance therapist Virginia Dryansky writes: "Based on contact with the concrete reality of the body, the strengthened ego can begin to replace delusionary thinking [with] percepts more congruent with reality."[10]

Art therapists sometimes claim that through art, which contains such opposites as action and contemplation, impulse and control, ways can be developed to deal with patients who are unapproachable with words.[11] However, the overwhelming use of the arts therapies in the treatment of psychotic patients has been reported anecdotally in case histories. Much has been written in the form of hypothetical conjecture — that is, what *should* work. A good deal of work remains to be done in the experimental validation of the assertions of practitioners.

In music therapy, in which much more experimental work has been conducted, treatment claims tend to be more modest and narrow. As a result, the use of music therapy in the treatment of psychotic patients rests on a more solid footing, but is also confined to clearly adjunctive and ancillary functions. A major function seems to be that of socialization.

The neurotic, or "anxiety," disorders, as they increasingly have come to be called, are of a quite different nature from schizophrenia or from the severe mood diseases. First of all, they are often disorders of the so-called "normal neurotics" in our society. On the one hand, those who suffer neuroses are often not readily identifiable from their overt behavior or their language. On the other hand, those suffering more acute neurotic disorders may exhibit some of the symptoms of psychotics; not too long ago, neuroses were sometimes called "minor psychoses." Increasingly, however, therapists have come to question whether neuroses — at least in their milder forms — are really illnesses.

The fears, concerns, and anxieties of the neurotic are, for the most part, mental "distresses" rather than mental "illnesses." The major difference seems to be the ability of the neurotic to take control and to snap back. Many behaviorists, especially, see neurotic behavior as learned "maladjustive" behavior that can be unlearned; in fact, the majority of neurotic symptoms are subject to "spontaneous remission" — they tend to disappear by themselves. Moreover, current thinking distinguishes psychotic and neurotic behaviors by pointing to the fact that psychotic behavior is accompanied by — and perhaps caused by — clearly identifiable biological changes.

Comparing neurotic depression and psychotic depression, Dr. Peter Whybrow, dean of the Dartmouth Medical School, thinks that the psychotic has suffered a fundamental physiological and neurochemical change that prevents him from snapping back. "It's as if all the circuits [of the central nervous system] were overloaded somehow," he says, "and everything were bouncing back and forth in there."[12] And, unlike the psychoses, the neuroses are less likely to be of an either-or quality. They involve a continuum of distress from mild anxiety, which is normal and even essential to human functioning, to the disabling fears, compulsions, or depressions that may interfere with normal functioning.

The impatience with pain and discomfort that has characterized our age has resulted in a remarkable expansion of the concept of mental disorder, far beyond the core of the brain dysfunctions. The American Psychiatric Association's *DSM III*, the revised *Diagnostic and Statistical Manual* adopted in 1980, cites as treatable disorders: "tobacco-use disorder," "caffeinism," and shyness and malingering; and the "life problems" with which psychotherapists may grapple range from marital incompatibility to job dissatisfaction and boredom.

The growth of the concept has had two major results. One is the development of the tranquilizer era, characterized by the widespread marketing of drugs designed to alleviate even the most trivial manifestation of anxiety, depression, or unhappiness. Psychiatrist Leslie H. Farber claims that a major consequence of the trivialization of drug use is the abdication of personal responsibility:

> Accepting responsibility is hard and painful. [Patients] used to say: "It's not my fault. My parents did it to me. I'm only this way because of my childhood, my race, my poverty, my riches, my schooling, my sex, the shape of my nose." Now they say: "It's not me. It's a biochemical disorder in my brain." And they can prove it, because there's a pill that will make them feel better.[13]

Perhaps not, Farber concludes. No pill on earth, he contends, will make anyone better; there are only pills that will make people *feel* better. Mental health, he asserts, transcends symptomology.[14]

The other result of the impatience with unhappiness is the spectacular growth of what have come to be called "the helping professions." A phenomenon that is at the same time a cause and a result of this growth is the switch in support for at least the top echelons of this field from the individual to third parties — insurance companies, Medicare, Medicaid, Blue Cross and Blue Shield, and CHAMPUS for military dependents. According to critic E. Fuller Torrey, the growth of the tranquilizer industry has turned psychiatric hospitals into places where pills can be dispensed quickly and efficiently by trained nurses,[15] thereby freeing psychiatrists for work with the growing number of neurotic help-seekers. But the psychiatrists are not only too few in number to cope with the tide of anxious and unhappy supplicants, they are too expensive for many. So an army of workers has mobilized that includes clinical psychologists, psychotherapists, social workers, psychiatric nurses, school psychologists, guidance counselors, encounter group leaders, sensitivity group facilitators, peer counselors, an ill-defined category of "rehabilitation counselors," and a myriad of teachers of self-help programs ranging from assertiveness training and transcendental meditation to rebirthing and hot-tub therapy.

In the pushing, shoving, and elbowing for position in the treatment of the shady side of the human condition, the emerging arts therapies are struggling to define their roles. Indications are emerging that, in some areas at least, they can accomplish what other therapies — including the verbal psychotherapies — cannot, or that they can accomplish them better, or that they can add significant dimensions of accomplishment.

Because of the generally acknowledged medical nature of mental illness — madness — the treatment of the insane has been preempted by psychiatrists, who may enlist the aid of clinical psychologists (generally assigned to testing and diagnosis) and to a host of "adjunctive" therapists, including arts therapists. While much of the actual treatment is medical (pharmacological), the theoretical orientation of most workers in mental hospitals, from psychiatrist to adjunctive therapist, is predominantly psychoanalytic, except in the case of music therapy, in which a heavy behaviorist bias is deemed compatible with medical treatment.

In contrast, the treatment of the neurotic is an open field into which have poured, from every conceivable theoretical persuasion, practitioners of a bewildering variety of methods and techniques. The growing demand for experimental validation in the therapies offers promise that only those therapies that can support their claims with research findings will flourish and that the novelty and gimmick approaches will — if not disappear — be relegated to the soft fringes of the therapies.

FUNCTIONS OF THE
ARTS THERAPIES

By and large, despite the clear differences between those who suffer madness and those who suffer neurotic, or anxiety, distresses, the functions of the arts therapies seem to cut across the distinctions.

Diagnosis

The issue of diagnosis in mental health is a highly controversial one in which psychiatrists, social workers, civil liberties groups, and lawyers have been engaged in swirling dogfights.

In 1979, the American Civil Liberties Union and the Children's Defense Fund brought before the Supreme Court (and lost) a case that challenged the power of parents and psychiatrists to have children committed to mental institutions, to perform operations on them, and to administer drugs to them without the due process that would be accorded an individual accused of murder. The groups argued that it is incredibly easy for parents to "doctor shop" for a psychiatrist willing to commit a child on a diagnosis that might well be questioned by other psychiatrists. Indeed, given the disagreements in the field of mental health over diagnostic labels, it is possible to find vigorous disagreements over the diagnosis of any individual by qualified and trained experts.

Obviously, diagnosis in mental health is a subject that should be approached with considerable care by any therapist, verbal or nonverbal. Indeed, many in the therapies oppose the whole notion of diagnostic labeling—that is, assigning someone to a category like schizophrenia or manic-depression. "Diagnostic labels are dangerous," writes Walter Kempler. "They are like glue, they flow on readily and must be peeled off slowly bit by bit."[16] Not only do they confuse the patient, he says, but they influence others who deal with the patient, and, "worst of all, they impair the vision of the therapist who makes them. . . . The only reason for diagnostic labels that I can find is to treat the anxiety of the therapist."[17]

To many—especially those who adhere to the medical model in the treatment of personality disorders—diagnostic labels are a useful device for categorizing individuals, a shorthand to help the therapist ascertain appropriate treatment. Critics, however, point out that the categories can easily become pigeonholes in which patients are filed so that the therapist can relieve himself or herself of the hard decisions about appropriate personal treatment.

Actually, general categorical labels are not often very helpful, apart from indicating the type of drug to be administered in cases of severe illness. Certainly, in the case of reactive disorders—those that are clearly responses to environmental influences—very few individuals who have been described with the same label are enough alike to benefit from identical treatment. The labels do not usually help the therapist to see through to the individual's problems, handicaps, or circumstances so that the treatment may be appro-

218

priate to the person. Moreover, the definitions are often too vague to be useful in diagnosis. Dr. Robert Spitzer, who presided over the revision of the American Psychiatric Association's manual, acknowledges the fuzziness of the definitions in the old manual. He told an interviewer:

> Take schizophrenia. They'd mention delusions, hallucinations, thought disorder, impairment in social relations, flattening of affect, and so on. But you never knew whether some or all of these had to be present before you made the diagnosis. They didn't specify because it's easier to be vague.[18]

In contrast with the three pages of criteria in *DSM II* for diagnosing schizophrenia, the 1978 proposed revision of *DSM* had almost twenty, in an attempt to avoid ambiguity. However, the storm of criticism that has raged over the revisions since they were first unveiled as proposals in 1975 suggests that uniformity in diagnosis is not likely even among psychiatrists in the near future.

Arts therapists undoubtedly are influenced in their work by the diagnostic labels that are applied to patients by psychiatrists and psychologists, but perhaps less so than are verbal therapists, because much of the diagnosis in the arts therapies is independently derived. In fact, the diagnostic data collected by art therapists and dance/ movement therapists are often used to corroborate the psychiatric clinical diagnosis. Both art production and movement can reveal much about personality idiosyncracies. A patient can participate in either without formal training. Indeed, to the degree that a patient has been trained in either art or dance, the therapist faces the problem of distinguishing between "authentic" production, or response, and the conditioned response that reflects the training itself. This distinction is less a problem among the severely disturbed than among neurotic patients; the mental illness itself not only disintegrates the personality, but shows itself in distortions even among patients with prior training.

Diagnosis in the two fields is quite similar in some respects: for example, distorted body image may suggest psychosis. In some ways, though, diagnosis in the two fields is quite different. A patient who draws a picture produces an actual image—a direct source of diagnostic data for many therapists—that bypasses the intermediate step of translation into words. For most persons, however, drawing is not a common or usual activity, and the product may have what psychometricians would call "restricted content validity"; in other words, it may not reflect the patient's total personality—only his or her state of mind at the moment. In addition, it is a function of the patient's willingness to cooperate in the activity. Dance/movement, in contrast, uses as its diagnostic instrument that constant betrayer of the inner human, the body; movement is less susceptible to deliberate distortion or suppression.

But dance/movement may reveal less about abnormalities that are not actually psychotic. Art therapist Edith Kramer contends that there is no art form in which the relationships between style, development, and personality are as pervasive and clear as in the visual arts. "In the performing arts," she insists, "conditions are less absolute. For example, schizophrenia influences body movement . . . but the movement of psychopaths [those who can form no emotional attachments, who exhibit no signs of social responsibility, and who often become habitual and unrepentent criminals, usually referred to today as sociopaths] is not usually hampered by their illness, and it would not be possible to draw inferences about their disturbance from their dance."[19]

Each therapy, of course, has its diagnostic limitations. For example, while movement and stance are continuous and therefore present a greater range of content than does drawing, the movements themselves are fleeting and must often be captured for analysis by a notation system, itself an intermediate symbolic language.

For the most part, diagnosis in both art therapy and dance/movement therapy is based on traditional psychoanalytic categories; suggestive symptomologies that are pegged to such categories have been developed by some therapists in both fields. Central to psychoanalytic theory is the concept of the unconscious as a key to human behavior; in both art therapy and dance/movement therapy, spontaneous productions provide peepholes into the unconscious. They may reveal patterns and syndromes that are suggestive of specific mental illnesses and disorders. Consequently, such "authentic" production is highly prized in both therapies by practitioners who are psychoanalytically inclined. Interestingly enough, spontaneous production is also valued by humanist practitioners, but—since so many humanists reject not only psychoanalytic theory, but the medical model as well—for reasons that have little to do with diagnosis. To many humanists, spontaneous or authentic production is itself therapeutic and self-fulfilling; it is a step toward individuation.

In both therapies, nonspontaneous approaches are also used for diagnostic purposes. In the visual arts, patients may be asked to produce work within narrowly defined limits, or even to interpret images that have already been produced. The purpose of limiting response is to allow for the standardization of reactions; responses can be categorized and labeled. Such standardization is preferred by many behavioral therapists who distrust the primarily clinical (nonexperimental) approach of psychoanalysis, as well as the individual-centered approach of the humanists.

In dance/movement therapy, nonspontaneous production might include the use of set or patterned dances, such as folk dances or even waltzes. Many therapists who are psychoanalytically inclined frown on the use of such "nonauthentic" work on the ground that it is not revealing. Some go so far as to reject accompanying music that might introduce extraneously prompted, emotional cues to movement. Those dance/movement therapists who do use nonspontaneous approaches usually do so for reasons of opportunity rather than as a matter of diagnostic choice. They find that in some situations, resistant patients who find threatening the idea of spontaneous movement are willing to participate in patterned group dances. However, even in the performance of set dances, much is revealed about individual idiosyncracies.

Both art and dance/movement may be valuable sources of diagnostic data, but both are susceptible to facile oversimplification. Writing about the difficulties in diagnosing from spontaneous production in art, Nolan D. C. Lewis warns:

> Without a special technique in the hands of a trained investigator it is difficult or practically impossible to judge what mechanisms are represented when they are incorporated in a complicated drawing. . . . Psychologically we are dealing with complex problems in which each factor must be segregated, analyzed, studied, evaluated, and then brought again into relationship with the total situation.[20]

Little evidence can be found in the literature of music therapy to suggest the use of music for diagnosis. What little has been published is more concerned with response *to* music than with the production *of* music. Because of the indirect nature of such responses, and because of the need to translate emotions and responses into words, music listening seems to hold little promise for diagnosis. Two possibilities suggest themselves: the application of diagnostic techniques to spontaneous production that requires no training (such as humming or singing); and the measurement of purely physiological responses. (The latter has been done frequently in music therapy, but for other than diagnostic purposes.) However, little interest in the development of such diagnostic approaches is evident, and the possibilities remain hypothetical.

Interpersonal Relations

One major function common to all the expressive arts therapies is the encouragement and development of better interpersonal relationships and the sharpening of interpersonal communication. The specific objectives and approaches, however, vary sharply in the different arts therapies. In the visual arts, for example, the focus is on the therapeutic situation itself, on the communication between patient and therapist, and on the relationship between the two. Except in the relatively young field of family art therapy, there seems to be little interest in the development of relationships independent of the therapeutic setting.

In sharp contrast, a major concern in music therapy is socialization *between* patients. Music therapists tend to view music as a "social" art, and they stress its value in reintegrating the individual into a social situation. A major objective is that of drawing the individual out of himself, improving his relationships with others, and fostering group activity and group cooperation. This emphasis is very much in line with the social adaptation bias of behaviorism, and it is expressed in helping the individual to function as a member of a group.

Dance/movement therapy, like music therapy, is concerned with resocialization. The view of movement as communication and as interpersonal contact is tied up with the concept of interactional synchrony. Central to the concern with interpersonal communication are the concepts of "body language" and of culturally influenced movement conventions. It is the recognition of these signals and qualifiers and disclaimers that enable individuals to perceive and interpret nonverbal messages accurately.

Because both music therapy and dance/movement therapy are concerned with establishing or reestablishing human bonds, it is not surprising that some of the techniques are similar. Most striking, perhaps, is the use of "mirroring" techniques with autistic children and schizophrenic adults. In both, the device of picking up, or mirroring, rhythms or movements is designed to establish empathetic bonds with such patients as a way of breaking the barrier of isolation, of establishing interactional synchrony, and of building a basis for meaningful interpersonal relationships.

Catharsis

This function is common to both art and dance/movement therapies; it centers on the need of individuals to release tensions and to *express* their emotions, rather than the need to *communicate* with others. In dance/movement, the body itself acts as the instrument for the release of tension, but the fact that such release is often accompanied by fantasy testifies that it has psychic as well as physical elements.

Many therapists believe that the expressive act in itself may be healing as well as relieving—this view seems to be more common among art therapists than among dance/movement therapists. Many in both fields, however, see catharsis as temporary relief that is useful mainly in making patients more receptive to further therapy. In both therapies, moreover, catharsis is often an incidental or a concomitant function in many activities that are designed for other purposes.

Catharsis, in the same sense, does not seem to be a major function in music therapy. Neither in the classic Gaston work nor in any of the other major works in music therapy do the words "catharsis" or "release" appear in the index. The discussion of tension release is couched in behavioral terms; music therapists prefer to talk of response to stimuli—either stimulating or sedative music—to which responses are usually described in terms of physiological changes, such as reduction in tension levels or contractions, and changes in gastric motility.

Personality Integration

Integration is a psychoanalytic term that has gained wide acceptance among humanists. It can probably be understood best by contrasting it with *dissociation*.

Those who suffer from dissociative neuroses have not been able to resolve conflicts or reconcile their deep-seated feelings with reality. The essence of dissociation is a splitting of the personality, so that the repressed feelings are driven underground where they need not be tested against the realities of the outside world. Children's fantasies are a prototype of dissociation. The boy who has been reprimanded by an adult may conform outwardly but may create a private fantasy world in which—like a comic book hero—he vanquishes villainous adults or proves his superiority by coming to the aid of helpless, bungling adults.

Such dissociation is natural among children, but it is considered abnormal for adults. Among the forms of dissociative neurotic behavior are amnesia (loss of memory, in which an individual blocks out intolerable experiences), sleepwalking (in which unconscious wishes are transformed into actions while the superego is relaxed), and a complete change of personality (in which an individual may go "berserk," or otherwise act out repressed impulses). Extreme forms of dissociation may involve the complete disintegration of the personality and a flight from reality into a fantasy world.

Integration involves "reality testing"—that is, the attempt to find solutions to problems by trying them out in the real world, and with real people. Whereas dissociation is passive and private, integration involves active participation with others. To existentialists, dissociated personality elements are *non*self, *non*being, *non*entity, while the integrated personality *is* the self. Integrative experiences involve recognition of the buried conflicts and repressed feelings and the reconciliation of the unconscious with the conscious. The concept of integration focuses on *balancing* the elements of play, fantasy, and dreams with the constraints of reality.

In light of the heavy behaviorist orientation in music therapy, it is understandable that integration does not appear frequently in the literature of the field. Phenomena that are not overtly and directly observable—like repressions, or even the unconscious—are not to be taken seriously in behaviorism. To many music therapists, therefore, the integrative function has no meaning. Even those who recognize the existence of an unconscious are uncomfortable unless they can face the manifestations of the working of the unconscious in the form of behavior; it is the behavior with which they deal, not the unconscious.

In sharp contrast, the integrative function plays a prominent role in both art therapy and dance/movement therapy, and it is a central concern alike of psychoanalytically oriented practitioners and humanist therapists.

In the visual arts, both Freudian and Jungian therapists see a basic function of therapy in promoting a dialogue between the conscious and the unconscious. To do this, they seek to explicate and interpret the symbols and dream images that are messages from the unconscious. Doodling, in particular, is sometimes viewed as a valuable technique both for diagnosis and for bringing to the surface previously hidden elements of the unconscious.

Dance/movement therapists who are psychoanalytically inclined may encourage free, authentic movement on the part of a patient as a technique for bringing into the open repressed emotions and feelings, which can then be tried out in the world of reality.

Many practitioners in both therapies believe that it is not enough merely to bring elements of the unconscious to the surface, but that a two-fold affective-cognitive approach is necessary in order to help the patient sort out the ambiguous and often misunderstood feelings that bubble up. In both therapies, therefore, expressive work (somatic or productive) often includes or is accompanied by cognitive work; arts therapists often work in teams with verbal psychotherapists, or themselves become "arts psychotherapists."

In both therapies, humanist practitioners view the integrative function in terms of holistic approaches, the purpose of which is broader than mere therapy and is applicable to all individuals. In this vein, the humanist who talks of "integrating experiences" or of gestalt art "experiences" rather than "therapy" is dealing with a broad self-improvement model, the goals of which are interrelatedness and closure rather than healing in the medical sense.

THE EXPRESSIVE ARTS THERAPIES AND EDUCATION IN THE ARTS

Expressive arts therapists are perennially concerned with distinguishing between arts therapy and education in the arts. The dividing lines are not always clear in terms of what is actually done in each. Though a good deal has been written on the subject, the answers can best be described as equivocal. In part, this is the result of disagreements on the theoretical level.

The arts themselves have always evoked emotional response, and both education in the arts and the arts therapies are concerned with emotion. One unresolved question in which much of the debate centers is whether "aesthetic" and "associative" responses can be isolated. Roger Fry asserts that they can, suggesting that the distinction between art education and art therapy must rest on such a discrimination.[21] Fry writes: "The form of a work of art has meaning of its own and the contemplation of the form in and of itself gives rise in some people to a special emotion which does not depend upon the association of the form with anything else whatever. . . . The esthetic emotion is an emotion about form."[22]

Fry admits that the majority of people view works of art in terms of associated emotions, memories, ideas, symbols, and images. He contends, however, that works of art in which appeal rests mainly on such associated emotions rarely survive the generation for whose pleasure they were made, while those works that emphasize only order and purely formal relationships have a curious vitality and longevity in art. "In proportion as an artist is pure," he says flatly, "he is opposed to all symbolism."[23]

Similarly, Henri Focillon contends that form represents only itself and is primary. When it is allied with symbolism, he claims, "form is tortured to fit a meaning."[24] Focillon goes further than Fry and argues that our very perception of the world is shaped by "the logic of the eye, with its need for balance and symmetry,"[25] a logic that is not always in agreement with the logic of structure.

On the other hand, many psychotherapists, and not a few art therapists, tend to view all art processes as servants of underlying urges, wishes, memories, and conflicts. Some, especially among the psychoanalytically oriented, deny the existence of an aesthetic or creative urge that is independent of other, more basic, urges and drives. Freudians, for example, tend to attach sexual significance to artistic production. Theorist Anton Ehrenzweig writes: "Man neutralized his sexual urges and guilts with esthetics. . . . I follow Freud in assuming that the esthetic pleasure transmuted a sexual (visual or acoustic) voyeurism."[26]

Such exclusively sexual interpretations of artistic production invite the scorn of many non-Freudians. Jungian therapist Herbert Read writes that in Ehrenzweig's view, "all works of art are but species of fig leaves."[27] Read himself prefers to see art—particularly among children—as expression of conflicts at the levels both of the personal unconscious and the collective unconscious; the latter, Read calls "the wellspring of art." Mandalas, in particular, are images of wholeness and integration.[28]

Some believe that while all art production may have a psychological basis, it is possible to distinguish aesthetic from other expressive elements. Ernst Kris thinks that art is fundamentally communication between the artist's id and his ego under the "protection of the esthetic illusion."[29] Kris suggests that the essence of aesthetic production is conscious communication rather than self-expression.[30]

Implicit in most distinctions between art education and art therapy is the concept of aesthetic creation. To most therapists, the aesthetic element (no matter how it is defined) is the province of the art educator, and the "associative" elements are the concern of the art therapist. In operation, the distinction is not always clear. Moreover, some art therapists argue that successful art therapy *must* focus on the aesthetic; the artistic value of a work of art, contends art therapist Edith Kramer, is a measure of successful sublimation, and therefore of therapeutic success.

Possibly, the most generally accepted distinctions between education in the arts and in the arts therapies are based on the purposes of the activities. In music, in which education and therapy converge more closely than in the other arts, Gaston sees purpose as the key to the distinction. He writes that music therapy and music education are much more similar than is commonly realized. Certainly, the good music educator adheres to the basic principles of music therapy, and the good music therapist applies the practices of music education. He concludes:

> Perhaps music therapy and music education can best be distinguished by the fact that the music therapist is chiefly concerned with eliciting changes in behavior, not with perfecting musical endeavor. . . . The music therapist is more sensitive to the non-musical behavior of the child, the music educator to the musical behavior of the child. Even so, music therapy and music education have much in common.[31]

In music, particularly, the distinction between education and therapy is made more difficult by the fact that in most settings, a prerequisite to, or a concomitant of, the therapeutic use of music *is* music instruction; patients are usually taught to play instruments or to sing in groups.

Claire Schmais, director of the dance therapy program at New York's Hunter College, thinks that dance teachers and dance therapists engage in clearly distinguishable role relationships with their subjects. A dance teacher who focuses on a child's oedipal complex, or a dance therapist who spends the therapy session teaching the fine points of a *tour jeté*, would be violating her professional role. It is the purpose of the activity, she claims, not the nature of the client, that identifies the role:

> Both teacher and therapist may work with the same clientele, e.g., the retarded, the blind, the deaf, etc., but this does not alter their role definitions. Dance teaching does not become therapy because the clientele is handicapped or in need of therapy. A profession is not defined by whom it serves but by what it does. A dentist treating an emotionally ill patient is doing dentistry, not dental therapy.[32]

In this view, a dance teacher would have no qualms about imposing a style or a technique (such as Graham modern dance technique) or a movement (such as contraction) because the dance itself, including style and technique, is at the heart of the process. In contrast, a dance therapist must guard against imposing a style that overlays and covers the patient's expression.

The distinction is not absolute. Jungian art therapist H. Irene Champernowne thinks that teaching techniques and skills is compatible with the goals of therapy, as long as such teaching does not dominate "the drive to creative expression." Playing with fantasy is the basis for both creative expression and the process of therapy. Nevertheless, Champernowne insists, there *is* a difference, and she contends that much of the "art therapy" practiced in institutions is actually art education, or even recreation:

> Far be it from me to deprecate any of the work done to lighten and enrich the time spent by people in hospitals, prisons, and schools of various kinds. . . . But therapy is more than passing time: it is healing in depth and if *therapy* is to become harnessed to a partner called *art*, there is a great danger that art will override the partnership, because for some it is more exciting and has greater appeal. It has results to show and does not, as true therapy must, *necessarily* force the "teacher" or "therapist" into an often uncomfortably deep involvement with sick or suffering individuals.[33]

In all of the arts therapies, humanist practitioners tend to blur the distinctions between art education and art therapy, or dance education and dance therapy. Since they reject the psychoanalytic medical model, many such practitioners reject also the term "therapy." Thus, humanist Janie Rhyne prefers the term "gestalt art experience" to "art therapy," apparently seeing little difference between the encouragement of self-actualization in an educational or in a therapeutic setting.[34] Mary Lee Hodnett claims that while psychoanalysis serves amply for diagnostic purposes and even for communication, "to bring a patient's art therapy to an end without encouraging, coaxing, prying for, or insisting on finding his artistic creativity is once again to serve only part of a meal."[35] She continues:

> Encourage patient clients to draw pictures in the service of helping you to see and interpret their problems if you must, but don't stop there. As your patient grows in insight and tries to shift himself into more realistic and fruitful ways of thinking and consequently, of behaving, give him also the thrill and satisfaction of finding his own uniqueness in and through art.[36]

It should be noted that such humanistic art therapists do not entirely blur the distinction between art as therapy and art education. Hodnett urges practitioners to make no value judgments in terms of currently accepted art standards in their dealings with patient products. However, if the principles of self-actualization and individuation were to be applied consistently in setting goals for humanistic education, then we might reasonably expect that a humanist art *teacher* would accept the same *caveat*.

A recurrent theme in all the literature of the arts therapies, and one that cuts across all of the psychological compartmentalizations, is the point that the primary difference between art education and art therapy rests on role and purpose. In art education, the teacher's task is to help the student develop creativity or technique *as an artist;* in art therapy, the practitioner's major responsibility is to help the client develop *as a human being.* Technique in art education refers to *artistic* technique; in therapy, it refers to technique for promoting change in personality.

INTERRELATIONSHIPS
BETWEEN THE ARTS THERAPIES

A major theme of this book is the contention that the expressive arts therapies share some fundamental assumptions about the value of nonverbal expression and communication in the treatment of individuals. Such shared assumptions are manifested in common concepts, goals, and functions. For example, distortions in body image will be expressed differently in drawing than in movement but experienced practitioners in both art therapy and dance/movement therapy should agree on the nature and extent of the distortion and in their assessments of the implications.

There is some evidence that the arts therapies share more than theoretical constructs (often derived from one or another psychotherapeutic theory) and diagnostic concepts. An intriguing relationship seems to exist, at a very fundamental level, between the various senses themselves, a relationship that has only recently been subjected to serious analysis.

Observers have long noted a strange connection between our responses to sensory stimuli. We will often react to a stimulus (like the color *red*) in terms of another sense (*hot*), or in terms of a temperamental characterization (*excitable*), or in terms of meaning (*energy*). Experimental studies have shown that subjects will respond to sound tones as bright or dark, rough or smooth, sweet or sour, heavy or light, hollow or full; even single notes have been shown to cause changes in muscular tension.[37] One experimenter found that for children, patterns of tones and musical selections are significantly related to geometric patterns and colors.[38]

The assignment of meaning to sensation is probably most obvious in the area of color: an individual's physical health may be color coded (he may be in the pink, or he may be wan), and emotions are often described in colors: green (with envy), blue (with melancholy), red (with rage). As a result, the investigation of "meanings" in sensations has tended to concentrate in the area of color perception.

According to art psychologists Hans and Shulamith Kreitler, there are five types or dimensions of such meanings:[39]

1. *Body expression* (blue is constrictive and binding).
2. *Sensations and feelings* (blue is cold).
3. *General abstraction* (blue is spiritual, although, if carried to an extreme, it may be moralistic, as in "blue laws").
4. *Metaphoric* (blue is like the world beyond).
5. *"True symbols,"* in which contrasts and solutions are presented simultaneously (blue is a fusion of heavenly peace and the destructive fire of lightning).

Many color associations, of course, are culture biased. Some relationships are so common, however, and cut across cultures to the degree that they have been conventionalized and generalized. And many of these associations are so generally shared that they have an almost universal quality.

In the search for the roots of these shared associations, psychologists of the arts have investigated the phenomenon of *synesthesia*, the crossover of responses in terms of alternative senses. The bulk of the studies, as in the search for meaning, has focused on color associations. Some of the more common synesthetic experiences involve: *temperature* (reds, oranges, and yellows are experienced as warm, while blues and greens are cool); *weight* (dark colors like black or brown are heavy, while whites and yellows are light); *size* (brightly colored objects seem larger than dark or dull objects); and *distance* (blue advances and red recedes; on the other hand, the sharper the contrast between the color and its background, the closer it appears).[40] This crossing over of sensations can be experienced in a variety of ways, and color can be evoked by odors, sounds, tastes — and even numbers. The phenomenon of "color hearing" has been noted frequently; individuals will often see colors when they listen to sounds, especially music.[41]

Synesthesia has been confirmed in laboratory experiments, and — as might be expected — conflicting hypotheses have been advanced to explain the phenomenon. Behaviorists tend to be most impressed by those studies that suggest a physiological basis. Stimuli of temperature, taste, odors, electrical stimulation, chemicals, and even tilting of the head all seem to promote changes in sensitivity to specific colors. Conversely, changes in illumination enhance tactile sensation and sensitivity to sounds.

Color consultant Faber Birren notes that in addition to sensation crossover, colors affect the neuromuscular system: reds tend to increase bodily tension and to stimulate the autonomic nervous system, while greens and blues release physical tension.[42] The physiological hypotheses seek a connection, as yet unidentified, between the brain's various sensory centers. However, the same experimental finds are cited by humanists to support an "organismic" or "holistic" hypothesis, based on the conjecture that an individual responds as a whole to any stimulus, rather than as a series of parts. As far back as 1939, an experimental study demonstrated that color affects movements, varieties of sensations, and a subject's general emotional attitude; one conclusion was that reds and yellows are "expansive" colors that involve the individual with the world, while blues and greens are colors of "contraction" and "concentration."[43]

While psychologists are intrigued with the phenomenon, little has been done to work it into any of the theories of personality or into any of the practices of psychotherapy. Despite the obvious implications for their work, synesthesia has been largely ignored by arts therapists on a practical level, and few studies have been conducted by arts therapists in intersensation reactions with a view to building a joint or common theoretical structure. Part of the problem may be the fact that arts therapists tend to have approached their practices from the narrow base of theory in one therapy and proficiency in one underlying art. They tend to see themselves as specialists rather than as generalists in the arts. In addition, most therapists see themselves as practitioners rather than theoreticians. As a result, most of the meaningful research in this area is being done by psychologists of the arts, who are more interested in theoretical considerations than in practical application.

Some hopeful signs have emerged that there is an increasing convergence of the arts therapies in some areas, and it is likely that such convergence may eventually spur both interdisciplinary and multidisciplinary research. Increasingly, training programs for arts therapists have come to recognize the shared assumptions and the common bases of the arts therapies. Some provide for common core courses for all arts therapists; others encourage interdisciplinary and multidisciplinary programs, even for therapists who will receive degrees in one specific therapy. At institutions like Hahnemann Medical College in Philadelphia, therapist-teachers in the various disciplines plan and work together. In 1974, the training programs for arts therapists were reorganized at Hahnemann to provide for common core experiences.

At about the same time, art therapist Myra Levick and dance

therapist Dianne Dulicai began to experiment with joint family analyses and evaluations. The first joint evaluations were conducted in simulated class experiences with their own students; the approach was extended to work with medical students, inservice staff, and the staffs of other training centers. Levick and Dulicai write:

> It became more and more apparent that the joint approach to looking at families and the system in which they were operating, and joint observations of individual members within the family, provided data far more complete than a single evaluation process. It also became apparent that while certain sophisticated cognitive skills could seem to be more representative of ego strength, the body movement notated by Mrs. Dulicai seemed to indicate the degree to which the individual was defending against primitive impulses; [these analyses] reinforce and support data collected from family drawings in defining the family system.[44]

The development of joint assessment practices may presage joint research projects into such phenomena as synesthesia and, perhaps, to the development of intersensation theory applicable to the practice of the arts therapies.

Signs are emerging that techniques used in the arts therapies have begun to cross over between the therapies. For example, the *Draw-A-Person Test* by Karen Machover, frequently used in art therapy as a diagnostic tool, has begun to appear in the literature of dance/movement therapy as a measure of the change in body image that might result from movement therapy.[45]

THE DRIVE TOWARD PROFESSIONALIZATION

A major thrust in all of the expressive arts therapies is the drive to gain professional status in mental health. While practitioners have been referring to their occupations as professions, this designation has not been universally accepted by the dominant psychotherapists or by the public at large.

Probably the major immediate problem is the fuzziness of the definitions in the arts therapies and the boundaries of the practices. What are the functions of the expressive arts therapies? What are the recognizable techniques that differentiate them from the clearly adjunctive therapies like occupational therapy or physical therapy, on the one hand, and the psychotherapies, on the other? At present, the practitioners in the arts therapies have not been able to identify what they do or the purposes of their practices in terms that are acceptable to many in the neighboring fields (such as occupational therapy and special education) or in the psychotherapies.

The preoccupation with defining the arts therapies emerges in the newsletters, the journals, and the conferences. "How Do We Define the Parameters of Our Profession?" ask dance/movement therapists.[46] Art therapists are concerned with "Defining the Field"[47] and with "Problems of Definition."[48] Hodnett writes: "We will have to woo and soothe the psychiatrists, convince the thorny practicing artists that we are not in competition with them, threaten art educationists enough to make them seek to unite with us—at least with a view to having us let most of their territory alone."[49]

The term "profession" relates to a concept whose attributes are not clearly defined or universally accepted. In our technological society, occupational groups strive toward professionalization for purposes of status and income. As a result, a large group of occupations exist whose members call themselves professionals, but who are judged by others to be something less. Sociologists refer to such indeterminate groups by a variety of designations, some with positive, some with negative, connotations: semiprofessions, service professions, helping professions—and pseudoprofessions. For example, teachers, nurses, and social workers, who normally refer to their own callings as professions, are frequently viewed by outsiders as semiprofessionals. In the eyes of some observers, the remarkable preponderance of women in these fields has been a factor in hindering the struggle for professional acceptance.[50]

The commonly accepted attributes of a profession constitute a base in a substantial body of knowledge, a lengthy training period, exclusivity, and control over its members as well as over entry into the practice.

The drive toward professionalism in the arts therapies has been evidenced by the establishment of increasingly rigorous educational requirements for "registry," which, in all of the arts therapies discussed, includes an internship period. In dance/movement therapy, the fieldwork-internship is to be followed by a lengthy period of "supervised," full-time, paid employment as a dance therapist. Of the three arts therapies treated in this book, the least rigorous requirements obtain in music therapy, perhaps because this is the area in which proficiency in the underlying art itself is the most easy to ascertain.

In all the arts therapies, too, the national organizations have established codes of ethics and hope to have their registry requirements eventually become requirements for government licensure to practice. In the meantime, the evolving and increasingly exclusive requirements are the subject of bitter debate within the organizations themselves.

The internship requirement, particularly in dance therapy, is the subject of considerable concern. Internship is the subject of letters-to-the-editor pages of the ADTA *Newsletter*, articles in the organization's *Journal* (the recent establishment of which is itself seen as a move toward professionalization), and debates at sessions of the annual conferences. Some practitioners have been working in dance therapy for years and may have contributed to the growing body of knowledge in the field, but have chosen, for a variety of reasons, not to join the ADTA or to accede to the organization's code of ethics. Should licensure ever develop, they contend, the ADTA standards undoubtedly would be the basis for licensing, and they might effectively be frozen out of practice. Since the organization already provides for "equivalent" requirements, the real thrust of their objections is probably one of ideology. Implicitly or explicitly, each of the therapies has come to lean on the philosophical structure of one of the psychotherapies. Moreover, these ideological and practical affiliations are reflected in the educational and membership requirements of the national arts therapies associations.

For example, the internship requirements for ADTA registry call for work with psychotics at medical facilities—presumably to provide a broad-based experience for working with abnormal clients. However, virtually all of these facilities are psychoanalytic in approach, and these are the institutions in which neophyte therapists gain the bulk of their firsthand experience. Such restrictions have prompted vigorous criticism from both humanistically inclined practitioners and from some, like pioneer dance therapist Blanche Evan, who have chosen to work with neurotics. Evan, a charter member of the ADTA, pointed out in an open letter to ADTA members that her own work with "normal neurotics" for a generation would not be considered legitimate dance/movement therapy for registry purposes.

Professionalization of any practice is marked by an increasing awareness of the need to substantiate the claims of the practice. Especially in art therapy and in dance/movement therapy, the journals and proceedings have been filled with articles and papers that have tended to be highly theoretical (and often remarkably pedantic), and filled with terminology borrowed from medicine, or that have presented anecdotal data to bolster outcome claims. Only the *Journal of Music Therapy* has been research oriented, apparently because the behaviorist approach is well suited to experimental validation. In recent years, increasing numbers of articles have been appearing that point out the need for a rigorous research base to support the assertions of arts therapists and their claims to professional status. To date, few solidly researched studies have appeared, but there are indications that in the near future an increasing volume of experimental research will be reported in the journals of all the organizations.

In the area of outcome studies, two directions become immediately apparent. The major thrust is in the area of measuring psychological or attitudinal changes that may be attributed to the therapy. However, some practitioners confine their investigations to the behavioral changes that can be observed in the immediate area of treatment. For example, a dance/movement therapist might seek ways of ascertaining the degree to which movement therapy helps patients improve their body images or their self-esteem. Another might be concerned with merely notating and measuring change in effort/shape patterns or in movement repertoire.

The problem in the measurement of psychological change is the fact that such measurement must be inferential. We can measure such change only indirectly, by observing behavior. By and large, outcome research in this area is likely to employ the techniques that have developed in measuring the results of psychotherapy. They include:[51]

1. Assessment interviews, with a growing reliance on the use of standardized interviews to boost interjudge reliability.
2. The use of standardized personality tests like the MMPI, to measure changes in specific traits.
3. Behavioral assessment, using either inventories of specific symptoms (like the Fear Survey Schedule), or the use of checklists by observers.
4. Self-concept measures, used to report subjective distress.
5. Factor-analysis batteries.
6. Peer ratings, especially those used to score anxiety and specific behaviors.

The whole area of outcome study design is still in its infancy, and it is likely that significant advances will occur in this field that will help to provide feedback on the efficacy of therapy.

EXPANSION OF THE ARTS THERAPIES
INTO THE COMMUNITY

Until recently, the treatment of emotional and mental problems was generally associated with institutionalization. Several factors have combined to force rapid and drastic change, not only in our concept of treatment, but in the concept of mental health itself.

The goals and objectives of mental hospitals have changed, partly as a result of economic pressures, partly because of new developments in pharmacology and a change in thinking about the mentally ill. The skyrocketing costs of long-range hospitalization and the development of tranquilizers and antidepressants have made obsolete the old custodial function of state mental hospitals. Increasingly, these large state institutions have tended to become centers of intensive, relatively short-term therapy; they are custodians only of the dangerous or the helpless. This deinstitutionalization was spurred by a 1975 Supreme Court decision that ruled that patients could not be detained against their wills unless they were dangerous or unable to survive in the world outside. Most patients have been returned to their communities, in which local mental health centers are expected to provide not only emergency and inpatient care when needed, but training and rehabilitation to help patients obtain jobs.

The policy of localizing mental health care was enunciated in 1963 federal legislation that provided help in building community facilities and was bolstered by research findings that long-term commitment and the resultant social isolation only aggravate mental and physical deterioration. As a result, the population of state mental hospitals fell sharply, from 559,000 in 1955 to 193,000 in 1975—a drop of more than 65 percent.[52] The bulk of the patients has been dispersed to community mental health centers and to the private agencies and care centers that have proliferated.

The dispersal suggests that arts therapists may need to think increasingly in terms of short-term support programs with rapidly shifting patient populations. In community centers, the overriding long-range goal has come to be the building of socialization skills, and short-term objectives have come to focus on such obvious "coping" skills as self-care, interpersonal communication, and "behavioral control." To some, the change in mental health care may presage a significant shift from the long-term psychoanalytically geared programs in the arts therapies to an increasing focus on humanist here-and-now orientations and on the development of clearly

236

defined behavioral objectives to be achieved through practical behavioral methods. The extended programs may survive intact only in the residential care facilities and in private practice, particularly in the treatment of neurotics.

Unfortunately, as a team of *Newsweek* writers phrased it in 1978, "the bright hope for a new era in mental health has dimmed. True, many of the state hospital wards stand empty. But vast numbers of their former inmates are worse off than they were before."[53] In too many cases, communities have been unwilling or unable to provide the necessary financial and moral support to maintain the centers. In poorer communities, many simply do not consider financial support of mental health facilities a major priority; in many affluent communities, citizens are often afraid of dropping property values and violence in the vicinity of such facilities, and many are simply unwilling to acknowledge the existence of widespread mental illness in their midst. In some cases, the private agencies that have filled the void have had little interest in the area of mental health care beyond the profits to be made from federal support programs and have created what the *Newsweek* team called "miniature snake pits [that] have sprung up throughout the U.S. to exploit the newly released mental patient."[54]

It is true that the publicly supported and the nonprofit programs include some examples of mental health care at its best. The Cambridge-Somerville Center outside of Boston consists of forty facilities, including two halfway houses, three day care clinics, and a cooperative housing project and is staffed by a team of young professionals and paraprofessionals. The Fountain House Foundation in New York is a cooperative day care program that provides services for 1,200 former inmates while they live with their families, in licensed single-occupancy homes, or in foundation-owned apartments in scattered locations; it maintains a newspaper, runs a thrift shop, and maintains training programs.

However, in too many communities, the public-spirited citizens who administer the programs display more zeal than informed judgment; many are not knowledgeable enough to distinguish between trained mental health workers (including arts therapists) and the well-meaning but generally untrained volunteers who are anxious to help in the communities. Faced with constant financial pressures, these administrators often staff their centers on the basis of cost rather than expertise. As a result, many of the support programs have been activity programs rather than therapeutic ones: what passes for art therapy, dance therapy, and music therapy are frequently recreation programs. At this point, it is too early to ascertain whether the community programs must of necessity involve a diluted view of the arts therapies, or if the rampant volunteerism is a passing phase during a period of transition.

We noted earlier the expansion of the concept of mental health that has coincided with the remarkable growth of the use of drugs for the alleviation of mental distress and with the equally remarkable growth of the "helping professions." One of the outgrowths of the revolution of rising expectations in mental health is the mushrooming of a host of self-growth and self-improvement movements, often grouped under the rubric of humanism. Many of these groups are thought of as "therapies," despite the fact that most of them reject the medical model and tend to view therapy and self-improvement as virtually synonymous. Mary Lee Hodnett presents this expanded concept of the arts therapies:

> There is a better way to regard the arts therapist than as a servant of psychiatry. He is rather a member of the humanistic tradition that strives toward the upper reaches of man's potentiality. The expressive therapies are not mere tools for bringing subnormal behavior and poor mental health back to something resembling the norm. They constitute part of the highly cooperative effort needed to reach the upper levels of human functioning no matter how far down in the psychotic levels you must start. We must get away from the illness model and use a broader definition. We see the life cycle as central, and we view man as conducting his life with purpose.[55]

Humanist therapists have long sought to replace the hospital-based approach to therapy with a community-based one. The humanist view of community arts therapy is quite different from that on which the community mental health centers are based. In the latter, the hospital medical model has been modified to fit the confines and the limitations of the community centers. Disdaining the medical approach, humanists tend to encourage the expansion of nonverbal and creative arts therapies into a broad educational program. The result is a growing network of community arts centers, community educational programs, workshops, institutes, and development centers, in which the essential elements of the arts therapies are geared to the needs of essentially "normal" individuals to help them achieve their unique potentialities as human beings.

A major spur to the expansion of the arts therapies into the field of education is Public Law 94-142. This federal act mandates free appropriate education for all handicapped children, aged three to twenty-one, in the "mainstream" of public schools. Many of these children previously had been institutionalized or had been excluded from schooling altogether. As a result of this act, school systems have been made responsible for locating, identifying, and evaluating all exceptional children and for providing educational programs for them. The multidisciplinary team approach that is mandated by Public Law 94-142 has brought into schools increasing numbers of professionals — including arts therapists — who had previously been thought of as mental health practitioners rather than as educators. A spin-off of this trend is the increasing interest in the principles and techniques of the arts therapies by teachers of special education.

Perhaps the ultimate expression of the use of the arts in the service of mental health is in the early detection and prevention of problems, an approach that cuts across ideological affiliation. Edna Salant, an art therapist at the National Child Research Center, a large private preschool in Washington, D. C., provides art therapy for children who are referred by teachers for behavior that may be indicative of problems—aggression or withdrawal, for example—or because there may be stress situations at home. Salant involves teachers and parents in the program, which she sees as "both preventive and therapeutic." Preventive art therapy, she is at pains to point out, is quite different from art education. "For one thing," she says, "the therapist, like the room, is *exclusively* theirs . . . [and] the children understand that this time with the therapist is for them to use as they wish," whether that be playing out or communicating repressed feelings. Salant distinguishes between primary intervention—the treatment of a healthy child when troubles are occurring but before they cause serious emotional disturbance—and later intervention—the treatment of a child's symptoms before they become established—but she sees both forms of intervention as preventive. By using art therapy in such ways, she concludes, "one can prevent more serious problems from developing in [the child's] future."[56]

Dr. Judith S. Kestenberg, of the Child Development Research Center in Sands Point, N.Y., uses movement notation to analyze the kinesic interactions between mothers and infants. "In a few weeks or months," she contends, "we can identify and prevent potential problems or correct existing ones that might require years of psychotherapy later in life, and we can do much of it even before the child begins to speak."[57] The preventive function is a major concern of the child development centers that have been springing up in communities across the country. Some are affiliated with community hospitals, some with county mental health boards and mental health centers, while many are independently organized and maintained, usually as nonprofit corporations.

The long-range result of the drive to bring the expressive arts therapies into the communities and to expand their functions may well be a closing of the circle and a return of the creative and expressive arts to their ancient role in the development of healthy, functioning human beings.

REFERENCE NOTES

1. Silvano Arieti, "New Views on the Psychodynamics of Schizophrenia," *American Journal of Psychiatry* 124, no. 4 (October 1967):453–57.
2. E. Fuller Torrey, "Tracking the Causes of Madness," *Psychology Today* 12, no. 10 (March 1979):91.
3. "Chemical Clues to Schizophrenia," *Science News* 112, no. 21 (November 19, 1977):342.
4. Silvano Arieti, "Roots of Depression: The Power of the Dominant Other," *Psychology Today* 12, no. 11 (April 1979):54.
5. Ronald R. Fieve, Julien Medlewicz, and Joseph L. Fleiss, "Manic-Depressive Illness: Linkage with the Xg Blood Group," *American Journal of Psychiatry* 130, no. 12 (December 1973):1355–935.
6. Herman Van Praag, et al., "Cerebral Monoamines and Depression," *Archives of General Psychiatry* 28 (June 1973):827–31.
7. Joseph J. Schildkraut, "Neurochemical Studies of the Affective Disorders: The Pharmacological Bridge," *American Journal of Psychiatry* 127, no. 3 (September 1970):134–36.
8. Arieti, "Roots of Depression: The Power of the Dominant Other," p. 92.
9. Ibid.
10. Virginia Dryansky, "A Case Study of a Chronic Paranoid Schizophrenic in Dance Therapy," in *Monograph No. 3*, American Dance Therapy Association (Columbia, Md.: ADTA, 1974), p. 101.
11. Elinor Ulman, "Therapy Is Not Enough," in *Art Therapy in Theory and Practice*, eds. Elinor Ulman and Penny Dachinger (New York: Schocken Books, 1975), p. 21.
12. Quoted in Maggi Scarf, "From Joy to Depression: New Insights Into the Chemistry of Moods," *The New York Times Magazine*, April 24, 1977, p. 32.
13. Leslie H. Farber, "Marketing Depression," *Psychology Today* 12, no. 11 (April 1979):64.
14. Ibid.
15. E. Fuller Torrey, "A Merger of Oil Filters and Ids," *Psychology Today* 12, no. 12 (May 1979):120–26.

16. Walter Kempler, "Gestalt Therapy," in *Current Psychotherapies*, ed. Raymond Corsini (Itasca, Ill.: F. E. Peacock, 1973), p. 275.
17. Ibid.
18. Quoted in Daniel Goleman, "Who's Mentally Ill?" *Psychology Today* 11, no. 8 (January 1978):37.
19. Edith Kramer, *Art as Therapy With Children* (New York: Schocken Books, 1971), p. 7.
20. Margaret Naumburg, *An Introduction to Art Therapy* (New York: Teachers College Press, 1973), p. v.
21. Roger Fry, "The Artist and Psychoanalysis," *Bulletin of Art Therapy* 1, no. 4 (1962):3-18.
22. Ibid., pp. 8-9.
23. Ibid., p. 14.
24. Henri Focillon, *The Life of Forms in Art* (New York: George Wittenborn, 1942), p. 13.
25. Ibid., p. 9.
26. Anton Ehrenzweig, *The Psychoanalysis of Artistic Vision and Hearing* (New York: George Braziller, 1965), pp. 257-58.
27. Herbert Read, *The Forms of Things Unknown* (London: Faber and Faber, 1960), p. 91.
28. Ibid., p. 197.
29. Ernst Kris, *Psychoanalytic Explorations in Art* (New York: International Universities Press, 1952), pp. 61-63.
30. Ibid., p. 254.
31. E. Thayer Gaston, "Music Therapy and Music Education," in *Music in Therapy*, ed. E. T. Gaston (New York: Macmillan, 1968), p. 292.
32. Claire Schmais, "What Is Dance Therapy?" *Journal of Physical Education and Recreation* 47 (January 1976):39.
33. H. Irene Champernowne, "Art and Therapy: An Uneasy Partnership," *American Journal of Art Therapy* 10, no. 3 (April 1971):142.
34. Janie Rhyne, *The Gestalt Art Experience* (Monterey, Calif.: Wadsworth, 1973).
35. Mary Lee Hodnett, "A Broader View of Art Therapy," *Art Psychotherapy* 1 (1973):77.
36. Ibid., p. 79.
37. Max Schoen, "Conclusion: Art the Healer," in *Music and Medicine*, eds. Dorothy M. Schullian and Max Schoen (New York: Henry Schuman, 1948, reprinted by Books for Libraries Press, Freeport, New York), pp. 401-02.
38. L. Omwake, "Visual Responses to Auditory Stimuli," *Journal of Applied Psychology* 24 (1940):468-81.
39. Hans Kreitler and Shulamith Kreitler, *Psychology of the Arts* (Durham, N. C.: Duke University Press, 1972), p. 69.
40. Ibid., p. 67.
41. Rudolf Arnheim, *Visual Thinking* (Berkeley: University of California Press, 1969), p. 111.

42. Faber Birren, "Color Preference As a Clue to Personality," *Art Psycho-therapy* 1 (1973):13.
43. K. Goldstein, cited in Kreitler and Kreitler, *Psychology of the Arts*, p. 111.
44. Myra Levick and Dianne Dulicai, "Evaluation of Family Systems Using Art Therapy and Movement Therapy Modalities" (unpublished), p. 2, reprinted in *Proceedings*, Seventh Annual Conference of the American Art Therapy Association, 1976 (Baltimore, Md.: AATA, 1976), pp. 24-25.
45. Sheila Beth Franklin, "Movement Therapy and Selected Measures of Body Image in the Trainable, Mentally Retarded," *American Journal of Dance Therapy* 3, no. 1 (Fall 1979):44.
46. *ADTA Newsletter* 12, no. 6 (October 1978):7, and unpublished position paper by the past presidents of the ADTA, 1976.
47. Mary Lee Hodnett, "Toward Professionalization of Art Therapy: Defining the Field," *American Journal of Art Therapy* 12, no. 2 (January 1973): 112-17.
48. Elinor Ulman, "Art Therapy: Problems of Definition," in Ulman and Dachinger, *Art Therapy in Theory and Practice.*
49. Hodnett, "Toward Professionalization of Art Therapy," p. 110.
50. Amitai Etzioni, ed., *The Semi-Professions and Their Organization: Teachers, Nurses, Social Workers* (New York: Macmillan, The Free Press, 1969).
51. Allen E. Bergin and Hans H. Strupp, *Changing Frontiers in the Science of Psychotherapy* (Chicago and New York: Aldine and Atherton, 1972), pp. 56-62.
52. *The New York Times*, March 19, 1978, IV, p. 10.
53. "The New Snake Pits," *Newsweek*, May 15, 1978, p. 93.
54. Ibid., p. 94.
55. Hodnett, "Toward Professionalization of Art Therapy," p. 117.
56. Edna G. Salant, "Preventive Art Therapy With a Preschool Child, " *American Journal of Art Therapy* 14 (April 1975):67-74.
57. Personal interview at the Child Development Research Center, June 8, 1978.

INDEX

243

DATE DUE